CAREER SUCCESS IN NURSING

Lois White, RN, PhD

Former Chairperson, Professor
Department of Vocational Nurse Education
Del Mar College
Corpus Christi, Texas

DELMAR

™

THOMSON LEARNING

Australia Canada Mexico Singapore Spain United Kingdom United States

DELMAR

THOMSON LEARNING ™

Delmar Staff:
Business Unit Director: William Brottmiller
Executive Editor: Cathy L. Esperti
Acquisitions Editor: Matthew Filimonov
Editorial Assistant: Melissa Longo
Sr. Developmental Editor: Elisabeth F. Williams
Executive Marketing Manager: Dawn F. Gerrain
Art/Design Coordinator: Connie Lundberg-Watkins
Production Coordinator: Catherine Ciardullo

Printed in Canada
1 2 3 4 5 XXX 05 04 03 02 01

For more information, contact Delmar,
3 Columbia Circle, PO Box 15015, Albany, NY 12212-0515

Or find us on the World Wide Web at http://www.delmar.com

Library of Congress Cataloging-in-Publication Data
White, Lois.
   Career success in nursing / Lois White.
     p. cm.
   Includes bibliographical references and index.
   ISBN 0-7668-3545-6
   1. Practical Nursing—Vocational Guidance. I. Title.
  RT62.W455 2001
  610.73'06'93—dc21

                                   2001042531

Contents

Preface

Career Success in Nursing is designed to be used near the completion of a nursing program as students begin to think about seeking employment as a nurse. The focus is on knowledge and skills related to actual work situations and the changes encountered when shifting from the role of student to that of employee. Job skills such as preparing a résumé, applying for a position, and preparing for an interview are explained in detail.

Organization

Career Success in Nursing consists of four chapters, appendixes, and a glossary.

- Chapter 1, Leadership, discusses leadership theories, styles, and skills. Task assignment, duty delegation, and care prioritization are also covered.
- Chapter 2, After Graduation, addresses the processes of examination and licensure. Computerized adaptive testing is described in detail. Suggestions for studying for the NCLEX® responsibilities for maintaining a nursing license, and employment opportunities are also presented.
- Chapter 3, Seeking Employment, identifies key points for preparing a résumé, cover letter, list of references, telephone call script, job application, interview, and thank you note and provides examples.
- Chapter 4, Workplace Transition, focuses on nursing team members and member responsibilities. Job expectations and responsibilities, including job description, policies and procedures, evaluation, and conflict and confrontation are also discussed.

Features

Each chapter opens with **Learning Objectives** to guide the reader's learning. **Key Terms** are listed to highlight terms with which the reader should become familiar.

Professional Tip boxes offer tips and technical hints to help the learner make the change from student to employee. A **Summary**, multiple choice **Review Questions**, and **Critical Thinking Questions** at the end of each chapter will help the student remember and use the material presented. **Web Flash!** boxes guide the student to the Internet for current information related to chapter content. The **References/Suggested Readings** and **Resources** sections provide the student access to the source of material in the chapters and a place to find additional information.

The **appendixes** provide sample résumés; addresses, telephone numbers, and Web sites for boards of nursing; definitions of abbreviations and acronyms; and answers to the review questions. The **Glossary** defines all the key terms in the text.

Acknowledgments

My sincere thanks to the entire team at Delmar who have worked to make this book a reality. Once again, Beth Williams, developmental editor, has provided guidance, humor, and attention to detail to keep the project on schedule.

To the reviewers, Sally Flesch and Melanie King-Gulliver, I say thank you for the time spent critically reading the manuscript and for the pertinent remarks and helpful suggestions.

A big Thank You to all who worked on this text.

About the Author

Lois Elain Wacker White earned a diploma in nursing from Memorial Hospital School of Nursing, Springfield, Illinois; an Associate Degree in Science from Del Mar College, Corpus Christi, Texas; a Bachelor of Science in Nursing from Texas A & I University–Corpus Christi, Corpus Christi, Texas; a Master of Science in Education from Corpus Christi State University, Corpus Christi, Texas; and a Doctor of Philosophy degree in educational administration–community college from the University of Texas, Austin, Texas.

She has taught at Del Mar College, Corpus Christi, Texas, in both the Associate Degree Nursing program and the Vocational Nursing program. For 14 years she was also chairperson of the Department of Vocational Nurse Education. Dr. White has taught fundamentals of nursing, nutrition, mental health/mental illness, medical-surgical nursing, and maternal/newborn nursing. Her career has also included 15 years of clinical practice.

Dr. White has served on the Nursing Education Advisory Committee of the Texas Board of Nurse Examiners and the Texas Board of Vocational Nurse Examiners, which developed competencies expected of graduates from each level of nursing. She maintains membership in the Texas Association of Vocational Nurse Educators, Sigma Theta Tau International, American Nurses Association, and the National League for Nursing.

Dr. White has been listed in *Who's Who in American Nursing*. She currently serves on the Vocational Nursing Financial Aid Advisory Committee for the Texas Higher Education Coordinating Board.

LEADERSHIP

LEARNING OBJECTIVES

Upon completion of this chapter, you should be able to:
- *Define key terms.*
- *Describe the five leadership styles.*
- *Outline the skills needed for effective management.*
- *Summarize the five rights of delegation.*
- *Explain factors that must be assessed in establishing priorities of care.*
- *Compare and contrast the roles of the registered nurse, licensed practical/vocational nurse, and unlicensed assistive personnel.*

KEY TERMS

accountability	delegation	management
assertiveness	democratic	participative
assignment	laissez-faire	situational
autocratic	leadership	time management

INTRODUCTION

By now you may have mastered the nursing process and demonstrated competency in many of the technical skills you will be required to perform on a daily basis. There are still other skills you will need in order to become competent in practice. These are the leadership skills that will allow you to manage yourself and others, delegate and prioritize tasks, and resolve conflicts and problems that may arise in the workplace. As a new graduate, you will not be expected to have yet mastered these skills; rather, they will develop as you progress in your career. This chapter introduces these leadership skills and provides insight into the working environment.

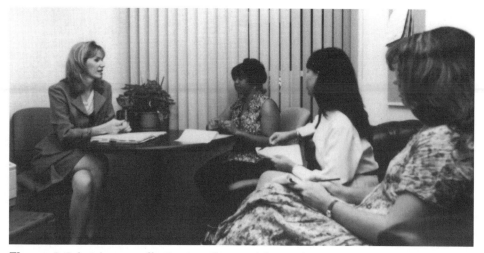

Figure 1-1 Leaders are effective in unifying and directing groups.

LEADERSHIP

Leadership is the ability to influence or motivate others to set and achieve goals. Many qualities are associated with leaders, such as creative thinking, self-direction, flexibility, excellent communication skills, and assertiveness. Leaders are considered critical thinkers, responsible decision makers, and role models. Leaders have a vision that directs a group and elicits the group's best efforts (Figure 1-1). Nursing leaders critically examine the way nursing care is delivered and use their power to effect change. Florence Nightingale, the prime example of a nursing leader, had a vision of what nursing should be, and her vision still guides nursing to this day.

Leadership Theories

Over many years, study and research have led to theories of leadership. These theories form the basis of thought about how a leader accomplishes work through the efforts of other people. The most commonly held theories include trait, contingency, path-goal, human relations, and transformational.

Trait Theory

The trait theory of leadership is the oldest. Leaders in government, the military, and industry were studied, and their traits were identified. Trait theory proposes that leaders are born with such traits as intelligence, initiative, drive, aggressiveness, and ambition and that these traits are related to being a successful leader.

Contingency Theory

The contingency theory of leadership looks at not only the leader but also the followers and the organizational perspectives (goals and objectives). The leader's effectiveness depends on the leader's style and the degree to which the leader controls and influences the outcomes. When the leader is matched with the organization's perspectives and the followers, the leader is very effective. When there is a mismatch among these three, leadership often is ineffective.

Path-Goal Theory

The path-goal theory describes an effective leader as one who assists the follower along the path toward a goal. This leader leads by coaching, providing guidance, and giving incentives that may not be customarily available. The leader reduces obstacles in the path of the follower toward the goal.

Human Relations Theory

Human relations theory focuses both on the leader and the followers with whom the leader interacts. The leader who understands the human element—needs, motives, and aspirations of others—and recognizes the other individuals' input is a successful leader.

Transformational Theory

Transformational theory applies to the leader who is able to bring out the best in others. Interactions between this leader and others are mutually uplifting and encouraging. Each party (leader and followers) inspires the others to greater achievement. This leader has charisma, provides idealized influence, intellectual stimulation, and inspiration and considers followers individually.

Leadership Styles

Several leadership styles are recognized. The style varies with the personality of the leader. Most often, a leader exhibits some characteristics of each style of leadership, though one style will typically be more dominant.

It is important to understand the various styles of leadership so you can identify and understand the approach of leaders and determine how to work most effectively with them. Also, it is important for you to have an understanding of your own predominant style of leadership. Knowing your style allows you to reinforce or alter it to enhance its effectiveness. Self-awareness about your predominant leadership style is the first step to being an effective leader.

Not all leadership styles are effective in all situations. Five styles of leadership are autocratic, democratic, laissez-faire, participative, and situational.

Autocratic

Autocratic leadership is task oriented and is based on the premise that the leader knows best. This leader is often viewed as controlling and inhibiting of the creativity and autonomy of workers. The leader solves problems and makes decisions without consulting the parties involved. All information is directed downward from leader to workers. The leader exercises responsibility for ensuring the work is done by issuing commands or orders to direct the work force and motivates others through praise, blame, and reward.

This leadership form is especially effective in crisis situations, in situations requiring a quick response, or when leading a group with limited knowledge. When workers have a certain degree of knowledge and teamwork is important, this style of leadership is not effective.

When working with an autocratic leader:

- Both praise and criticism are given.
- Instructions are clear and precise.
- Emergencies are taken care of quickly and efficiently.
- Workers seldom move beyond Maslow's level of safety in the work setting.
- *Never* get into a power struggle with this person.
- Participation in decision making does not occur.
- Qualities of caring are seldom exhibited. (Anderson, 2001)

Democratic

The underlying belief of the **democratic** style of leadership is that every member of the team should have input (Figure 1-2). Although democratic leadership is time consuming, the benefit is seen in increased cooperation and teamwork. This leader focuses on the individual characteristics and abilities of the workers and keeps in mind the commitment to whatever is best for the group. Individual workers are encouraged to participate in decision making and to express their viewpoints. The leader acts as a resource person and facilitator. This approach may not be effective when there is conflict within the group or when time is short. Problems occur when there is an emergency and there is no time for the group to process the information and come to a decision.

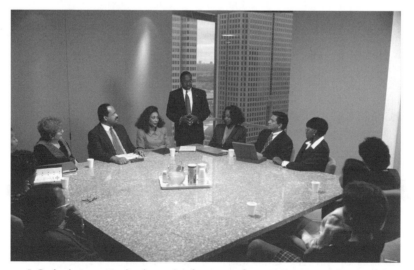

Figure 1-2 A democratic leader asks for input from the team during a brainstorming session. *(Courtesy of Photodisc)*

When working with the democratic leader:

- Each person is viewed as a unique individual.
- Individual needs are met when they do not interfere with the needs of the group.
- A time commitment is needed for the group process.
- Information and suggestions are freely shared with the group.
- Emergencies are stressful situations.
- Workers often move to the social and self-esteem levels on Maslow's hierarchy.
- Qualities of caring are exhibited. (Anderson, 2001)

Laissez-Faire

The **laissez-faire** leadership style is a passive, nondirect approach that gives leadership responsibilities to the group rather than to one person. Workers are without direction, supervision, or coordination. Praise, criticism, feedback, or information is not provided. The dissatisfaction level, which often is high, is caused by the lack of guidance, caring, and instructions. The group is often out of synchrony with the rest of the organization because information is not passed on to them. This style allows optimal autonomy and creativity for group members.

Task achievement is difficult under this leadership form, so it is not a style of leadership used frequently in health care. The leader is almost unidentifiable, relying on the group's strengths and initiative to accomplish tasks.

When working with the laissez-faire leader:

- Guidance, information, or individual attention is not provided.
- Autonomy and creativity are encouraged.
- Chaos is prevalent owing to lack of information.
- Synchrony with the organization is not present because information is not shared.
- Resentment toward the leader is evident.
- Workers seldom move beyond Maslow's level of safety in the work setting.
- Qualities of caring are not exhibited. (Anderson, 2001)

Participative Leadership

Participative leadership is a mix of autocratic and democratic styles. The participative leader makes proposals to the group, invites group criticism and comments, and then uses the feedback to make the final decision. Emergencies are handled immediately. Employees may freely share their ideas and contribute to the goal-setting process. This leader is confident in his or her own abilities and allows control and power to spread throughout the group.

When working with a participative leader:

- The work group has an active role in decision making.
- Information is shared with the group.
- There is a free exchange of ideas.
- Workers feel empowered.
- Workers are encouraged to function at the social and self-esteem levels of Maslow's hierarchy.
- Qualities of caring are generally exhibited. (Anderson, 2001)

Situational Leadership

Situational leadership depends on the situation, that is, the circumstances and people involved. Any or all of the previously described leadership styles may be needed in a particular situation. The effective leader identifies which style to use in the specific circumstance and which style to use with the individual persons involved.

Leadership Skills

Many theories of leadership cite several skills needed for *effective leadership*. These skills include communication, assertiveness, critical thinking, self-evaluation, and time management.

Communication

Strong communication skills foster trusting relationships with peers, subordinates, superiors, and clients, thus facilitating the leader's ability to motivate others. In addition, leaders must be able to convey ideas and information clearly, concisely, and persuasively to effectively implement changes in the delivery of nursing care.

Assertiveness

Assertiveness is a way of expressing oneself without insulting others (Hill & Howlett, 2001). Leaders communicate respect for the other person but not necessarily for the other person's behavior. The assertive leader is not aggressive toward other persons. By being assertive, a person claims responsibility for his or her own feelings, thoughts, and actions. Using *I* in statements shows that the person accepts responsibility for feeling, thinking, and doing.

Hill and Howlett (2001) suggest three rules for being assertive:

- Own your feelings. Do not blame others for the way you feel.
- Be direct in making your feelings known. Begin your statements with *I*.
- Be sure your nonverbal communication matches your verbal message.

Critical Thinking

Critical thinking skills incorporate the ability to analyze all aspects of a problem, explore options, find solutions, and implement changes. Critical thinking is a careful, deliberate process. Leaders seek information, consult experts, and use available resources to address problematic situations and to enhance care.

Self-Evaluation

The self-evaluation skills necessary for effective leadership involve an honest assessment of personal strengths and weaknesses. After such an assessment, efforts are made to enhance personal growth and development. An unwillingness to critically examine oneself hampers the leader's ability to critically examine situations, solve problems, and effect change in the workplace.

Time Management

Time management is a technique to help individuals get things done efficiently and effectively. It puts the individual in control. Leaders set goals, both long term and short term, to keep them focused. They set priorities for tasks to be completed and then see that the tasks are done the best way possible.

MANAGEMENT

Management and leadership are closely related concepts. **Management** is the accomplishment of tasks through the effective use of people and resources. Management involves the practical "nuts and bolts" of getting the job done with the available resources.

Nurses are in positions that require them to manage people and resources used to deliver quality client care. Managing the needs of a group of clients or managing the activities of a group of nursing assistants requires the same skills. Practice and education can help develop the management skills and, potentially, the leadership skills of every nurse.

As managers, nurses are expected to plan, organize, supervise, and monitor the care that is provided to a group of clients. The actual care may be accomplished by the nurse or by others, typically certified nurse assistants (CNAs) or some other type of unlicensed assistive personnel (UAP). Each aspect of management encompasses several components.

- *Planning:* identifying tasks to be accomplished, determining available resources, assessing skill level of workers, identifying problems, and setting priorities
- *Organizing:* making client assignments, ensuring availability of resources, sharing pertinent information, and determining time tables (e.g., of breaks, lunch, completion of certain tasks)
- *Supervising:* directing care provided by others, investigating problems, communicating information, reallocating people and resources as needed, and educating staff as needed
- *Monitoring:* determining whether tasks have been accomplished, assessing need for further action, and ensuring that appropriate documentation is completed

TASK ASSIGNMENT

An array of activities is involved in caring for clients, and all personnel have specific tasks they can facilitate. The ability of a specific staff member to perform a specific task is based on level of education and experience. Overlap exists, however, and determining who can legally do what is often confusing.

Tasks of the LP/VN

Registered nurses (RNs) and licensed practical/vocational nurses (LP/VNs) are individually licensed. Although some overlap exists in the scopes of practice of the

LP/VN and the RN, there are also some significant differences. Licensed practical/vocational nurses are dependent practitioners, meaning that an RN, doctor, dentist, or some other health care provider must supervise them. Most often the supervisor is an RN.

In addition to a scope of practice, LP/VNs and RNs have given scopes of competence. Within the scope of practice, there are tasks and responsibilities the individual may or may not be competent to implement. For example, it is within the scope of practice for the LP/VN to perform phlebotomy, but this task does not fall within the scope of competence of every LP/VN. The scope of competence expands as new skills are acquired, but all skills must fall within the scope of practice.

Licensed practical/vocational nurses are qualified to care for clients with common illnesses and to provide basic and preventive nursing procedures. Licensed practical/vocational nurses can participate in data collection, planning, implementation, and evaluation of nursing care in all settings. In most states, some specific activities are considered beyond the scope of practice of the LP/VN. These activities, with some variances by state, include the following:

- Client assessments (can collect data but not perform physical assessments)
- Independent development of the nursing care plan
- Triage, case management, or mental health counseling
- Intravenous chemotherapy
- Administration of blood and blood products
- Administration of initial doses of any intravenous medication
- Any procedures involving central lines

Tasks of the UAP

Nursing UAP do not have a scope of practice. A task that falls within the protected scope of practice of any licensed profession (including registered nursing and licensed practical/vocational nursing) *cannot* be performed by a UAP. These personnel can perform only those health-related activities for which they have been determined competent. These activities include the following:

PROFESSIONAL TIP

LP/VN Services

Any time nursing services are provided by an LP/VN, the supervising RN must be on the premises or immediately available by telephone. Being available by an answering machine or service does not fall within the definition of "immediately available." The amount of supervision is a function of the setting. In home health care or long-term care settings, it is common practice for the supervising RN to be available by telephone rather than on the premises.

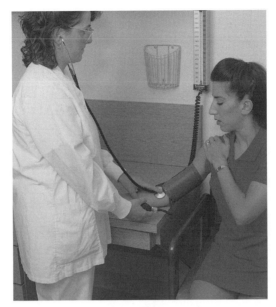

Figure 1-3 Unlicensed assistive personnel (UAP) can assist in many tasks, including measuring vital signs.

- Activities of daily living (feeding, grooming, toileting, ambulating, dressing)
- Vital signs (Figure 1-3)
- Venipuncture
- Glucometer use
- Mouth care and oral suctioning
- Care of hair, skin, and nails
- Electrocardiogram measurements
- Applying clean dressings without assessment
- Non-nursing functions (clerical work, transport, cleaning)

DUTY DELEGATION

Delegation is the process of transferring to a competent individual the authority to perform a select task in a select situation. State provisions for the delegation of nursing tasks vary. Some states allow for the delegation of nursing tasks by an RN to both LP/VNs and UAP. In some states, LP/VNs may delegate certain nursing tasks to other LP/VNs or to UAP. Other states restrict delegation to licensed personnel only. It is *most* important to know what is allowed in your state. The National Council of State Boards of Nursing Web site keeps a current listing of the address, telephone number, and Web address for each state board of nursing. This can be found at www.ncsbn.org.

The licensed nurse retains accountability for the delegation. **Accountability** is defined as responsibility for actions and inactions performed by oneself or others.

Assignment, another term frequently used to describe the transfer of activities from one person to another, involves the downward or lateral transfer of both responsibility and accountability for an activity.

At least one state differentiates between delegating nursing tasks to licensed nurses and assigning tasks to UAP. In New York, a nurse is not legally responsible for the process or outcome of care delegated to another licensed nurse. The nurse does remain responsible for tasks assigned to UAP, however. As an LP/VN, you are responsible for the decisions you make to delegate or assign tasks. Your knowledge of the client, activity, and worker will help you make sound decisions.

In most settings, RNs decide which nursing activities can be delegated or assigned to other licensed nurses (RNs or LP/VNs) and to UAP. Registered nurses and LP/VNs must consider five factors when making the decision to delegate or assign duties:

- *The potential for harm.* Certain nursing activities carry a risk for harming the client. In general, the more invasive a procedure, the greater the potential for harm. In addition, some activities carry a greater risk for certain kinds of clients (e.g., cutting the toenails of a diabetic). The greater the potential for harm, the greater the need for a licensed nurse to perform the activity.
- *The complexity of the task.* The cognitive skills and psychomotor skills needed for different nursing tasks vary considerably. As the skills increase in complexity, the level of education and competence becomes more critical. Some activities require a level of nursing assessment and judgment that can be provided only by a licensed professional.
- *The required problem solving and innovation.* As care is delivered, problems may develop. A successful outcome for the client may depend on a complex analysis of the problem and an individualized problem-solving approach. Alternatively, a simple activity may require special adaptation because of the client's condition. As problem solving increases in complexity and the need for innovation grows, so does the likelihood that a licensed nurse should provide the care.
- *The unpredictability of the outcome.* A client's response to an activity may be very predictable. If the client is unstable or the activity is new for the client, however, client response may be unpredictable and unknown. As unpredictability increases, so does the need for a licensed nurse.
- *The required coordination and consistency of the client's care.* Effective planning, coordination, and evaluation of client care require the nurse to have direct client contact. The more stable the client and the more common the medical diagnosis, the more the care that can be delegated to support personnel. The need for a licensed nurse increases as the required coordination needed to delivery quality care increases.

The five rights of delegation provide further direction in making appropriate decisions about delegation. They are as follows:

- *Right task.* The nurse must determine whether the task should be delegated for a specific client.

- *Right circumstance.* Factors to consider include the client setting, availability of resources, client's condition, and other factors.
- *Right person.* The nurse must ask the question, "Is the right person delegating the right task to the right person to be performed on the right client?"
- *Right direction/communication.* A clear, concise description of the task should be conveyed, including all expectations for accomplishing the task.
- *Right supervision.* Appropriate monitoring, implementation, evaluation, and feedback must be provided.

Registered nurses are frequently responsible for delegating care and assigning clients to the other nursing staff. In some settings, especially in long-term care settings, LP/VNs make these decisions. Licensed practical/vocational nurses should use the same guidelines to make decisions regarding delegating an activity to another LP/VN or assigning the task to UAP.

CARE PRIORITIZATION

Establishing priorities requires an understanding of the importance of different problems to the nurse, the client, the family, and other health care providers. For example, a client may be impatient to bathe because family is scheduled to visit. The nurse, however, does not want to remove the client's dressing for a bath until the physician has been able to examine the wound. Providing quality care while balancing such competing demands and ensuring completion of all tasks can be challenging.

Information obtained during the change-of-shift report is needed to appropriately establish priorities. This information can be useful in creating a worksheet identifying a list of tasks and target times for accomplishing these tasks. The time allotted for activities varies on the basis of the condition of the client, the availability of support personnel, the availability of supplies, and a number of other factors. The effective use of time is important whether caring for one client, caring for a group of clients, or supervising the activities of others providing care.

Although it is useful to get an overview of the day's activities, the clinical setting can change quickly and frequently, especially in acute care settings. The nurse must be flexible and continually evaluate and reorder the priorities of care.

Given the same assignment, nurses will not necessarily establish the priorities of care in exactly the same way. If working closely with an RN, you should determine the priorities as she views them. When supervising UAP, you must be clear about your priorities and expectations. Among the factors that can be examined when establishing priorities are the following:

- *Safety.* You should ascertain whether a safety situation must be addressed immediately. A client experiencing a cardiac arrest, a fall, an insulin reaction, and other situations presenting an imminent threat must be tended to first.
- *Timing.* Medications, tests, and vital signs are frequently ordered at specific times. Often, there is very little flexibility in shifting the times. In hospitals, medications, for example, must be given within a specified time frame, usually half an hour before or after the established time.

- *Interdependence of events.* You must ascertain whether some activity must occur before another activity can take place. For example, a fasting blood sugar must be completed before the client receives either insulin or food; blood is drawn a specified time after the medication is given to ascertain the peak level of gentamyacin.
- *Client requests.* Quality care depends on meeting client needs. Some events— showers, bed changings, enema administration, and so on—can be scheduled after consulting with the client regarding personal preferences.
- *Availability of help.* If two people are needed to turn a client, ambulate a client, or provide other care, coordination of the health care team is essential for effective utilization of time. Ascertain which activities require assistance, then consult with coworkers about their availability.
- *Client's status.* Clients vary in the extent to which they can participate in their care. This factor influences the order of executing tasks and the length of time a task takes. A semi-independent client can be performing a task (e.g., bathing) with minimal assistance while the nurse attends to some other need.
- *Availability of resources.* If six clients are supposed to get out of bed and sit in chairs, and only two chairs are available, the clients clearly cannot get out of bed at the same time. Geri-chairs, wheelchairs, and other equipment are sometimes limited. In addition, tasks may need to be delayed because supplies must be obtained from central supply.

Effectively organizing and establishing priorities with regard to care takes practice. Obtaining answers to certain questions when looking back at the day's events can help you hone this skill: Did you lack information that would have helped you prioritize more effectively? Did you fail to or inaccurately consider the client's status, the availability of help, or other factors? Did you establish priorities and set a schedule without getting client input? Did you fail to coordinate with coworkers? You must learn from experience. Both client and nurse feel the positive benefits of a day that flowed smoothly.

SUMMARY

- Common theories of leadership are trait, contingency, path-goal, human relations, and transformational.
- Leadership styles are typically classified as autocratic, democratic, laissez-faire, situational, or participative.
- Skills necessary for effective leadership include communication, assertiveness, critical thinking, self-evaluation, and time management.
- A good manager knows how and when to assign tasks, delegate duties, prioritize care, and resolve conflict.
- The decision to delegate a task should be based on the potential for harm, the complexity of the task, the problem solving required, the unpredictability of the outcome, and the required coordination of care.

- The five rights of delegation are the right task, the right circumstance, the right person, the right direction/communication, and the right supervision.
- Factors to assess when establishing priorities of care include safety, the timing of tests and other tasks, the interdependence of events, client requests, the availability of help, the client's status, and the availability of resources.

Review Questions

1. Pauline, an LP/VN, is the evening-shift charge nurse on 3B, a 40-bed unit in a long-term care facility. Christine is a CNA from another floor sent to work on 3B for the evening. She asks Pauline when she and the other three CNAs should take their lunch break. Pauline tells her to "work it out among yourselves." Pauline is using a style of leadership called:

   a. autocratic.
   b. situational.
   c. laissez-faire.
   d. participative.

2. The charge nurse discussed with all employees a proposed change for making lunchtime assignments and then, considering everyone's input, made the decision to keep things as they had been. This charge nurse was using a style of leadership called:

   a. participative.
   b. laissez-faire.
   c. democratic.
   d. autocratic.

3. The five rights of delegation include the right:

   a. person, task, time, and direction.
   b. time, task, person, and supervision.
   c. supervision, task, person, and direction.
   d. task, time, circumstance, and supervision.

Critical Thinking Questions

1. Nancy works in a long-term care facility as the evening-shift charge nurse on 4 West. One of her duties is to assign the CNAs to the clients. She also monitors their work and intervenes when necessary to ensure that clients receive safe and appropriate care. Lately, Nancy observes that Martha, a CNA, is not completing all her assigned responsibilities. How should Nancy address this problem?

⚡ WEB FLASH!

- Search the Web under broad categories such as *leadership, management, delegation,* and *employment.* What kind of sites do you locate?
- How is your search enhanced when you add qualifiers to narrow the search, such as *nursing, RN, LPN, LVN,* or *UAP?*
- Go to www.ncsbn.org; find and go to your state board's Web address. What do you find under delegation or nursing practice act?

References/Suggested Readings

Anderson, M. A., & Stolz, S. (2001). *Nursing leadership, management and professional practice for the LPN/LVN* (2nd ed.). Philadelphia: F. A. Davis.

Bernzweig, E. P., & Bernzwell, C. P. (1996). *The nurse's liability for malpractice: A programmed course* (6th ed.). St. Louis, MO: Mosby-Year Book.

Brent, N. J. (1997). *Nurses and the law: A guide to principles and application.* Philadelphia: Saunders.

Catalano, J. T. (1999). *Nursing now!: Today's issues, tomorrow's trends* (2nd ed.). Philadelphia: F. A. Davis.

Guido, G. W. (2000). *Legal and ethical issues in nursing* (3rd ed.). Englewood Cliffs, NJ: Prentice Hall.

Hansten, R. I., & Washburn, M. J. (1998). *Clinical delegation skills. A handbook for professional practice.* Gaithersburg, MD: Aspen.

Hill, S., & Howlett, J. (2001). *Success in practical nursing* (4th ed.). Philadelphia: Saunders.

Joint Commission on Accreditation of Healthcare Organizations. (1998). *Addressing staffing needs for patient care: Solutions for hospital leaders.* Oakbrook Terrace, IL: Author.

Loveridge, C., & Cummings, S. (1996). *Nursing management in the new paradigm.* Gaithersburg, MD: Aspen.

Marquis, B. L., & Huston, C. J. (1999). *Leadership roles and management functions in nursing theory and application* (3rd ed.). Philadelphia: Lippincott Williams & Wilkins.

Marriner-Tomey, A. (2000). *Guide to nursing management and leadership* (6th ed.). St. Louis, MO: Mosby-Year Book.

National Council of State Boards of Nursing. (1996). *Delegation: Concepts and decision-making process.* Chicago.

National Council of State Boards of Nursing. (1997). *The five rights of delegation* [On-line]. Available: www.ncsbn.org/files/uap/fiverights.pdf

National Council of State Boards of Nursing. (1999). *1998 profiles of member boards.* Chicago: Author.

Parkman, C. A. (1996). Delegation: Are you doing it right? *American Journal of Nursing, 96*(9), 43–47.

Swansburg, R. C., & Swansburg, R. J. (1999). *Introductory management and leadership for nurses* (2nd ed.). Sudburg, MA: Jones and Bartlett.

Trandel-Korenchuk, D. M. (1997). *Nurses and the law* (5th ed.). Gaithersburg, MD: Aspen.

Wilkinson, A. P. (1998). Nursing malpractice. *Nursing98, 28*(6), 34–38.

CHAPTER 2

AFTER GRADUATION

LEARNING OBJECTIVES

Upon completion of this chapter, you should be able to:
- *Define key terms.*
- *Explain computerized adaptive testing.*
- *Outline the steps to follow to take the NCLEX.®*
- *Compare and contrast various employment opportunities.*

KEY TERMS

computerized adaptive testing (CAT)
National Council Licensure Examination (NCLEX)

INTRODUCTION

You have completed the nursing educational program (Figure 2-1). Through formal education and clinical supervision, you have studied and learned the skills necessary to become competent in providing client care. Now you are ready to graduate and begin your career as a nurse.

Your first task as a graduate nurse is to take and pass the **National Council Licensure Examination (NCLEX®)**, an examination developed by the National Council of State Boards of Nursing that boards of nursing use in their licensure

PROFESSIONAL TIP

Temporary Permits
Although it may be possible to work during the period between NCLEX® testing and licensure, most employers will postpone hiring until after you have received your permanent nursing license. Therefore, do not be discouraged if you are unable to obtain employment as a graduate nurse during this period.

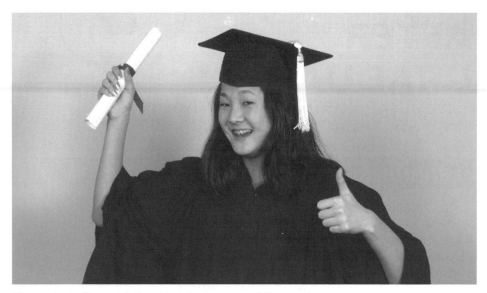

Figure 2-1 Congratulations! You have successfully completed your program.

decision making. The NCLEX-PN® is given to LP/VN candidates, and the NCLEX-RN® is given to RN candidates. There are many tasks to complete and skills to master to land your first job.

EXAMINATION AND LICENSURE

Examination and licensure are two separate processes that are usually applied for at the same time. The examination must be passed before licensure is granted. The examination uses computerized adaptive testing.

Computerized Adaptive Testing

Computerized adaptive testing (CAT) is a methodology for determining, by computer, a candidate's competence in the subject for which the candidate is being tested. The National Council of State Boards of Nursing (NCSBN) has identified the standard of competence for passing. All questions on the examination are classified by test plan area and level of difficulty. Questions are all multiple choice.

The test begins with a relatively easy question. If this is answered correctly, the next question the computer selects is more difficult. As long as the questions are answered correctly, the next question the computer selects is more difficult. When a question is answered incorrectly, the next question the computer selects is less difficult. Questions continue getting easier until a question is answered correctly, then the questions again become a little more difficult. This zigzag pattern continues until the candidate answers about 50% of the questions correctly (Figure 2-2).

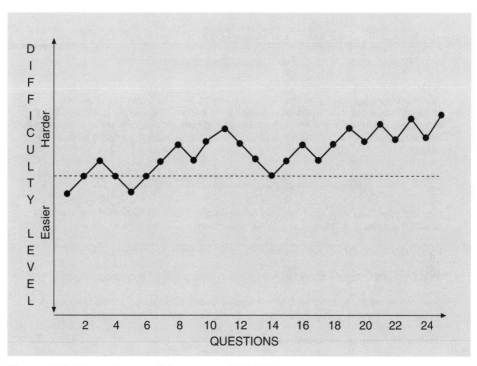

Figure 2-2 Zigzag Pattern of Answers on NCLEX.®

This represents the candidate's competence level. The computer selection of questions gives each candidate the best opportunity to demonstrate competence. A minimum number of questions must be answered.

Because everyone answers about 50% of the questions correctly, the difficulty of the questions answered correctly makes the difference in determining whether that candidate passes or fails. The pass/fail decision is based on the competence level corresponding to the difficulty of the questions, not on a percentage of questions answered correctly (NCLEX®, 2001).

Each candidate has a unique test (different questions and a different number of questions) based upon the answers given to the questions. The CAT is fair to each candidate, since all examinations follow the NCLEX-PN® or NCLEX-RN® test plan.

Knowledge, skills, and abilities essential for the safe, effective practice of nursing at the entry level for both LP/VN and RN candidates are tested on the NCLEX-PN® and NCLEX-RN®, respectively. Results of the NCLEX® are an important factor used by the various boards of nursing to make decisions about licensure. The NCLEX® is administered in all 50 states, the District of Columbia, American Samoa, Guam, the Northern Mariana Islands, and the Virgin Islands. Licensure endorsement from one board of nursing to another is facilitated because all boards of nursing use the same examination.

1. Apply to the board of nursing for a license, following instructions from that board.

2. Candidate receives an *NCLEX® Examination Candidate Bulletin* from the board of nursing.

3. Candidate submits a registration form and fee to the Chauncey Group (the National Council's contracted testing service) or registers by phone. The Chauncey Group will acknowledge the candidate's registration my mail. Fees are *not* refunded under any conditions. **Note:** Candidates seeking licensure from Illinois and Massachusetts do not register directly with the Chauncey Group. Follow registration instructions provided by those boards of nursing.

4. The board of nursing will communicate the candidate's eligibility to test to the Chauncey Group.

5. The Chauncey Group will send the candidate an Authorization To Test (ATT) with a booklet called *Scheduling and Taking your NCLEX®* Examination and a list of test centers.

6. The candidate will call a Sylvan test center and schedule an appointment to test.

7. On the appointed day, the candidate will take the test at a Sylvan Technology Center.

8. Sylvan transmits the test results to the Chauncey Group. After verifying the accuracy of the results, the Chauncey Group transmits them to the designated board of nursing.

9. The board of nursing sends results to the candidate.

Figure 2-3 NCLEX® Testing Process *(Reprinted courtesy of the National Council of State Boards of Nursing.)*

Figure 2-3 lists the steps each graduate must follow to take the NCLEX.® The contracted testing service changed in October 2001. Updated information can be found on NCSBN's World Wide Web site.

Results are mailed to the candidate by the state board of nursing 1 month or less after the examination. Candidates may retake the examination; however, the National Council requires a wait of at least 91 days between testings. Your state board of nursing may have other policies related to retaking the exam.

The NCLEX-PN®

The examination that all practical/vocational nurse candidates must pass in order to be licensed is the NCLEX-PN.® It follows a test plan based on the categories of Client Needs, which are:

- *Safe, Effective Care Environment*
  Coordinated care
  Safety and infection control
- *Health Promotion and Maintenance*
  Growth and development through the life span
  Prevention and early detection of disease

- *Psychosocial Integrity*
  Coping and adaptation
  Psychosocial adaptation
- *Physiological Integrity*
  Basic care and comfort
  Pharmacological therapies
  Reduction of risk potential
  Physiological adaptation

Integrated throughout the categories of Client Needs are concepts and processes fundamental to the practice of nursing. These concepts and processes are nursing process, caring, communication, cultural awareness, documentation, self-care, and teaching/learning.

This test plan looks very similar to the test plan for the NCLEX-RN.® They are both based on Client Needs. However, some of the subcategories are different, and the content included under each subcategory is different. For the entire test plan, go to www.ncsbn.org.

Candidates answer a minimum of 85 questions and a maximum of 205 questions during the maximum 5-hour testing period (National Council of State Boards of Nursing, 2001).

The NCLEX-RN®

The examination that all registered nurse candidates must pass in order to be licensed is the NCLEX-RN.® It follows a test plan based on the categories of Client Needs, which are:

- *Safe, Effective Care Environment*
  Management of care
  Safety and infection control
- *Health Promotion and Maintenance*
  Growth and development through the life span
  Prevention and early detection of disease
- *Psychosocial Integrity*
  Coping and adaptation
  Psychosocial adaptation
- *Physiological Integrity*
  Basic care and comfort
  Pharmacological and parenteral therapies
  Reduction of risk potential
  Physiological adaptation

Integrated throughout the categories of Client Needs are concepts and processes fundamental to the practice of nursing. These concepts and processes are nursing process, caring, communication, documentation, cultural awareness, self-care, and teaching/learning.

This test plan looks very similar to the test plan for the NCLEX-PN.® Some of the subcategories are different, and the content included under each subcategory is different. For the entire test plan, go to www.ncsbn.org.

Registered nurse candidates answer a minimum of 75 questions and a maximum of 265 questions during the maximum 5-hour testing period (National Council of State Boards of Nursing, 2001).

Studying for the NCLEX®

You have been preparing for this exam throughout your nursing program. Some review will probably be helpful. There are many review books on the market. The faculty may suggest one or two that they think are helpful. Several are listed in the References/Suggested Readings at the end of this chapter.

Most review books explain about the NCLEX® and computerized adaptive testing. The major part of the review book is made up of multiple choice questions covering all areas of the test plan. Correct answers and the rationale for each answer are usually provided. Some review books come with a computer disk or CD-ROM, so practice with a computer is also available. Many schools have computer lab times open for all students.

Be sure to read each question and all four answers carefully before choosing an answer. Try to eliminate one or two of the answers as incorrect. Then, if you have to, *guess*. By eliminating one or two of the answers, you will have a better chance of choosing the correct answer. Answer each question as it is presented. Do not skip a question and plan to come back to it. This strategy cannot be used on the NCLEX,® so practice now.

Plan the number of questions to answer during each study time so that all will be completed a day or two before you are scheduled to take the exam. Meeting this goal takes a great deal of self-discipline. Keep to your usual routine. Save the partying until after you have taken the NCLEX.®

Some schools have study groups to prepare for the NCLEX® that are facilitated by an instructor. Other schools may offer a short course on preparing for the NCLEX.® Commercial programs are also available, but these can be expensive. Choose the method for review that best fits into your schedule and way of studying.

PROFESSIONAL TIP

Taking the NCLEX®
- You must answer all questions as they are presented. You may *not* skip questions.
- If unsure of an answer, make your best guess and go on to the next question.
- Spend approximately 1 minute on each question.

Your License

After you have successfully passed the NCLEX,® you will be issued your nursing license from your state board of nursing. It is your responsibility to maintain your license according to your state's standards and to inform your state board of nursing of any changes in name, address, and employment. Once licensed, you are ready to practice.

EMPLOYMENT OPPORTUNITIES

A wide variety of employment opportunities exist, ranging from employment in the traditional settings of hospital and nursing home to less traditional settings such as home health care, residential care facilities, schools, government agencies, physicians' offices, or public health. In 1998, 692,000 LP/VNs were employed, with 32% in hospitals, 28% in nursing homes, and 14% in doctors' offices and clinics (Bureau of Labor Statistics, 2000a).

Employment in all settings for the LP/VN is expected to grow as fast as the average for all occupations through 2008. Physicians' offices, clinics, ambulatory surgical centers, and emergency medical centers are performing an increasing proportion of sophisticated procedures once performed only in hospitals. As health care generally expands, employment for the LP/VN is projected to grow much faster than average in these settings (Bureau of Labor Statistics, 2000a).

Although most LP/VNs are employed in traditional settings, increasing opportunities are arising in the nontraditional settings because of changes in health care delivery and nursing shortages.

In 1998, 2.1 million RNs were employed, with approximately 3 out of 5 RNs working in hospitals. About 1 out of 4 RNs worked part time (Bureau of Labor Statistics, 2000b). Employment for the RN is expected to grow faster than the average for all occupations through 2008. Although there will always be a need for hospital nurses, more positions will be found in home health, long-term, and ambulatory care (Bureau of Labor Statistics, 2000b). The nursing shortage will ensure employment opportunities in all areas.

An overview of various employment settings follows. As a graduate, it is your task to determine the setting that constitutes the best fit for you.

Hospitals

Although most LP/VNs work in the hospital setting, it is projected that the number of jobs for LP/VNs in hospitals will decline (Bureau of Labor Statistics, 2000a). Therefore, LP/VNs seeking to enter this setting will meet more competition than in the past. LP/VNs will typically find work outside of the client care unit, such as in hospital-based clinics, outpatient care units, and hospital-based long-term care units. Registered nurses will always be needed in the hospital. The area of growth for employment in the hospital will be in outpatient facilities such as same-day surgery, rehabilitation, and chemotherapy (Bureau of Labor Statistics, 2000b).

Long-Term Care Facilities/Rehabilitation Centers

Employment for LP/VNs in long-term care and rehabilitation settings is projected to grow faster than average (Bureau of Labor Statistics, 2000a). Long-term care will offer the greatest number of new jobs for LP/VNs because of the growing elderly population. Nurses in this setting will also provide care to clients who have been released by the hospital but who are not yet well enough to go home and who need additional rehabilitative services (Figure 2-4). Employment for RNs will also grow faster than average in this area (Bureau of Labor Statistics, 2000b). Most RNs are employed in administrative or supervisory positions.

Community Health Agencies

In the community health setting, care is provided to clients through established health care programs. These programs are generally funded by the local, state, or federal government or by voluntary agencies. Nurses in this setting generally work in a community clinic or travel to clients' homes to provide care and education.

Private Duty

Private duty nurses are self-employed, meaning the nurse is hired and paid directly by the client. Nurses work under the direction of a physician but must rely on their own knowledge and judgment to provide care. Private duty nurses are responsible for handling all matters of licensing and finances on their own.

Home Care Agencies

In the home care setting, care is provided to clients in their own homes. The nurse is generally employed by an agency but will work in the home of an assigned client. A much faster than average growth is expected in this area of nursing owing

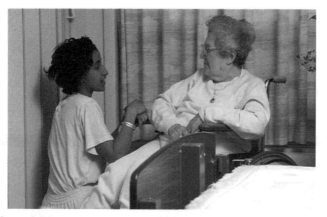

Figure 2-4 Care of elders in long-term care facilities is a growing career opportunity for the LP/VN.

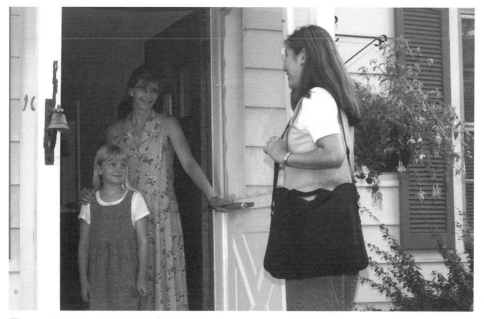

Figure 2-5 Nurses working for home health care agencies must travel to the client's home to provide care.

to both a consumer demand for home care and the lower costs of caring for an individual in the home (Figure 2-5).

Hospice

Hospice nursing care consists of providing comfort to dying clients and their families. The role of the nurse is to alleviate pain and other symptoms but not to provide curative care. The clients in the hospice setting are terminally ill and typically have fewer than 6 months to live. Hospice services are most often rendered in the home, but services can also be offered in other settings.

Occupational Health

Occupational health nursing serves to provide safe working environments in industrial workplaces. Occupational health nurses work within industries and corporations and collaborate with corporate administration to provide health education and promotion to employees in the workplace.

Correctional Facilities

Correctional nursing is the branch of nursing that provides care within prisons, youth detention centers, and probation divisions. Care provided ranges from ambulatory care to emergent care to comprehensive health care.

Schools

School nursing focuses on providing care to the school-age child. The school nurse serves to promote wellness and to identify or prevent problems. Both public and private schools offer opportunities for school nursing.

Parishes

Parish nurses provide health care education and support to a congregation. The care is designed to meet the common needs and beliefs of a specified group of people (Palmer, 2001).

Insurance Companies

Nurses working in the insurance setting are often responsible for coding treatments, providing physical examinations for insurance policies, and reviewing medical records.

SUMMARY

- Examination and licensure are two separate processes. The examination must be passed before licensure is granted.
- Each candidate receives a unique test based on whether the previous question is answered correctly or incorrectly.
- The NCLEX® test plan is the basis for all examinations. There are separate test plans for the NCLEX-PN® and the NCLEX-RN.®
- There are many employment opportunities for nurses.

Review Questions

1. On the NCLEX,® every candidate:

    a. answers 205 questions.
    b. spends 5 hours taking the test.
    c. receives test results within 1 hour.
    d. answers about 50% of the questions correctly.

2. The candidate who answers the minimum number of questions:

    a. failed the test.
    b. passed the test.
    c. either failed or passed the test.
    d. pushed an incorrect key on the computer.

3. Employment opportunities for the LP/VN are expected to decline in:

   a. hospitals.
   b. home care agencies.
   c. long-term care facilities.
   d. physicians' offices and clinics.

4. Employment opportunities for the RN are expected to:

   a. decline in hospitals.
   b. increase in home care agencies.
   c. decline in physicians' offices and clinics.
   d. remain the same in long-term care facilities.

Critical Thinking Question

1. The day before you are scheduled to take the NCLEX® there is a death in your family. How should you proceed?

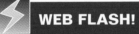

WEB FLASH!

- Search the National Council of State Boards of Nursing Web site (www.ncsbn.org). What information do you find? How can this be helpful to you?

References/Suggested Readings

Aliperti, L. (2000). *Licensed practical nurse exams* (Academic Test Prep). Lawrenceville, NJ: Arco Publishers.

Andreas, C. (2000). NCLEX-RN made ridiculously simple. Miami, FL: MedMaster.

Beare, P. (Ed.). (1999). *Davis's NCLEX-PN review* (2nd ed.). Philadelphia: F. A. Davis.

Beare, P., & Thompson, P. (Eds.). (1998). *Davis's Q & A for the NCLEX-RN*. Philadelphia: F. A. Davis.

Billings, D. (1998). *Lippincott's review for the NCLEX-RN* (6th ed.). Philadelphia: Lippincott Williams & Wilkins.

Burckhardt, J., Irwin, B., & Phillips-Arikian, V. (2001). *NCLEX-RN* (5th ed.). New York: Kaplan.

Bureau of Labor Statistics. (2000a). *2000–01 occupational outlook handbook. (Licensed Practical Nurses)*. [Online]. Available: http://stats.bls.gov/oco/ocos102.htm

Bureau of Labor Statistics. (2000b). *2000–01 occupational outlook handbook. (Registered Nurses)*. [Online]. Available: http://stats.bls.gov/oco/ocos083.htm

Curlin, V., Allen, H., & Sanchez, S. (2000). *How to prepare for the NCLEX-PN with CAT CD-ROM* (4th ed.). Hauppauge, NY: Barron's Educational Series.

Dahlhauser, M. (2000). *NCLEX/CAT-RN core review study guide.* New York: McGraw-Hill Professional Publishing.

Eyles, M. (2001). *Mosby's comprehensive review of practical nursing for NCLEX-PN* (13th ed.). St. Louis, MO: Mosby.

Frye, C. (2001). *Frye's 2500 nursing bullets for NCLEX-RN* (4th ed.). Springhouse, PA: Springhouse.

Mourad, L. (1998). *American nursing review for NCLEX-PN* (3rd ed.). Springhouse, PA: Springhouse.

National Council of State Boards of Nursing. (1998). *Test plan for the National Council Licensure Examination for Practical Nurses.* [Online]. Available: www.ncsbn.org

National Council of State Boards of Nursing. (2000). *Test plan for the National Council Licensure Examination for Registered Nurses.* [Online]. Available: www.ncsbn.org

National Council of State Boards of Nursing. (2001). *NCLEX candidate examination bulletin.* [Online]. Available: www.ncsbn.org

Palmer, F. (2001). Parish nursing: Connecting faith and health. *Reflections on Nursing LEADERSHIP, 27*(1), 17–19.

Saxton, D., Nugent, P., & Pelikan, P. (Eds.). (1998). *Mosby's comprehensive review of nursing for the NCLEX-RN* (16th ed.). St. Louis, MO: Mosby.

Silvestri, L. (2000). *Saunder's comprehensive review for NCLEX-PN.* Philadelphia: Saunders.

Silvestri, L., & Connor, M. (Eds.). (1999). *Saunders' Q & A review for NCLEX-RN.* Philadelphia: Saunders.

Smith, S. (2001). *Sandra Smith's complete review for the NCLEX-PN* (7th ed). Englewood Cliffs, NJ: Prentice Hall.

Springhouse. (1999). *Review for the NCLEX-RN: Questions & answers made incredibly easy, 3000+ questions* (10th ed.). Springhouse, PA: Springhouse.

Stein, A., & Miller, J. (1999). *Delmar's NCLEX-RN review* (4th ed.). Albany, NY: Delmar.

Timby, B., & Vaughans, B. (1998). *Lippincott's review for NCLEX-PN* (5th ed.). Philadelphia: Lippincott Williams & Wilkins.

Waide, L., & Roland, B. (1998). *The Chicago Review Press NCLEX-PN: Practice test and review book* (2nd ed.). Chicago: Chicago Review Press.

Zerwekh, J., & Claborn, J. (2000). *NCLEX-PN: A study guide for practical nursing* (3rd ed.). Dallas, TX: Nursing Education Consultants.

Resource

National Council of State Boards of Nursing (NCSBN), 676 North Saint Clair Street, Suite 550, Chicago, IL 60611-2921; 312-787-6555; www.ncsbn.org

SEEKING EMPLOYMENT

CHAPTER

3

INTRODUCTION

Seeking employment, for many people, is synonymous with scanning the Sunday want ads. This is not necessarily a bad place to identify potential employers; after all, an organization that is advertising is probably hiring. The problem with relying solely on this approach is that it limits you to the jobs that are available rather than the job you want. Many job openings are not advertised in the newspaper. Job vacancies exist well before they are advertised. Remember, using this method, you are in competition with all the other job seekers who are relying on want ads to identify employment options.

Other options exist for identifying potential employers. The telephone directory is a great place to identify health care facilities in your area. You are likely to find far more health care facilities in your local area than you ever imagined. All these facilities represent potential employers. Job counselors disagree on the usefulness of telephoning the employers to determine whether job vacancies exist: Some claim that a telephone call is a quick method of determining vacancies, whereas others believe a face-to-face visit to the facility yields better results.

A job club, perhaps formed with your nursing school classmates, is often an effective method of sharing information about employers, vacancies, job requirements, and the like. In addition, a job club can be a morale booster. Your colleagues in the club may also offer insights into those areas of nursing for which they believe you are most suited.

After you have identified potential employers, be persistent in your job hunt. Most important, go after any job that looks interesting to you regardless of whether there is a known vacancy. But don't stop there. Apply at many different organizations. Apply not just at *different* facilities but at *many* facilities. Concentrate on small employers. Every health care job seeker has heard about the local large medical center. However, right around the corner from your home may be the less well-known school for developmentally disadvantaged children, and waiting there may be your ideal job!

Potential employers can be identified in several other ways. Nursing journals typically advertise positions. Sometimes, your instructors know of positions. The state or local employment office may offer assistance. Professional job placement services are also available, but they usually charge a fee. Corporate Web sites often post job openings along with job-seeking information and tips (Smith, 2000). Try using your favorite search engine to find employment opportunities. Nursing jobs may be found at virtualnurse.com. Many places of employment are looking for and accepting electronic résumés.

You graduated, passed the NCLEX®, and were issued a license to practice. Now it is time to begin seeking employment. The job search requires up-front preparation on your part to organize and pinpoint the areas where you would like to concentrate your efforts. After graduation, take the following steps to secure a job:

1. Identify your objective.
2. Prepare a résumé.
3. Prepare a cover letter.
4. Prepare a list of references.
5. Prepare a telephone call script.
6. Complete a job application.
7. Prepare for the interview.
8. Prepare a thank you note.

IDENTIFY YOUR OBJECTIVE

A common mistake among persons seeking employment is identifying potential employers as a first step. Most employment counselors advise beginning the job search with *you*. Identify your job target or objective first. If you cannot envision yourself as a medication nurse in a long-term care facility, there is very little reason to apply for such employment in that setting.

Identifying your objective accomplishes two important things. First, once you know your objective, you will know where to focus your efforts in identifying potential employers. Second, you will have a reference point for deciding what to say about yourself on a résumé or during a job interview. You will be prepared to tell prospective employers precisely the ways that you can be of benefit to them.

If you are having difficulty pinpointing your objective, think back to other jobs or volunteer projects in which you have been involved. What skills did you use? What did you like about the job or project? List your strongest four to six skills: These are the skills that you want to use in your new job and that will be valuable in identifying your objective. Ascertain which jobs call for those skills. The skills needed for a particular job can be identified in a number of ways, including the following:

- Talking to people in nursing positions and asking them what they like and do not like about their jobs. During clinical in nursing school, you may have already talked to nurses and have more information than you realize.
- Reading the job descriptions in the classified ads.
- Calling places that employ nurses and asking them to send you a job description.

Once you have matched your skills to the skills required in a particular job, you have effectively identified your job objective.

PREPARE A RÉSUMÉ

The **résumé** is a job-hunting tool that summarizes your employment qualifications. The content of the résumé should be factual, accurate, and honest. The focus should be on verifiable skills or accomplishments that suggest what you can do for an employer who hires you. The résumé may be targeted toward a specific job, a specific career field (e.g., licensed practical/vocational nursing), or a specific person. Some employers want a résumé; others rely on job applications; and still others ask for both a résumé and a job application.

Essential Elements

Regardless of the format selected, the essential elements of a résumé include the following:

- *Heading:* name, address, telephone number, e-mail address (if you have one)
- *Objective:* the type of position you are seeking
- *Work experience:* job title, dates of employment, employer (with city and state), responsibilities, special projects, accomplishments; listed in reverse chronological order (most recent job first)
- *Education:* schools (with city and state), major (area of concentration), certificate or degree earned and date; listed in reverse chronological order; include high school if you did not attend college

In the course of developing your résumé, make a list of all your past jobs. A sample worksheet is provided in Figure 3-1.

WORK EXPERIENCE

Job One

Job Title _____

Dates _____

Employer _____

City, State _____

Major Duties _____

_____

Special Projects _____

_____

Accomplishments _____

_____

Job Two _____

Job Title _____

Dates _____

Employer _____

City, State _____

Major Duties _____

_____

Special Projects _____

_____

Accomplishments _____

_____

Figure 3-1 Sample Worksheet for Work Experience

Having significant gaps in your employment history may give the impression that you are an unstable worker. Employment gaps can be explained in a number of ways. If the gap resulted because you were in school, include that information. If you did significant volunteer work during that period, describe those activities. Being a full-time parent or a full-time caregiver to a family member is a respectable activity that sufficiently explains gaps in paid employment.

Similarly, make a list of your education. You certainly want to include training and education you have completed. A sample worksheet is provided in Figure 3-2. If you have completed only a portion of training, list the courses that are directly related to your objective. The same idea applies to college courses you may have taken. It is usually not necessary to mention a high school diploma, unless the position you seek calls for one or you have no other higher education.

EDUCATION

School _____

City, State _____

Degree _____

Major or Area of Concentration _____

School _____

City, State _____

Degree _____

Major or Area of Concentration _____

School _____

City, State _____

Degree _____

Major or Area of Concentration _____

Figure 3-2 Sample Worksheet for Education

Optional Elements

Other information may be important to include on a résumé. Worksheets similar to those in Figures 3-1 and 3-2 can be made to organize these optional elements. The optional elements of a résumé include the following:

- *Honors:* the name of the organization bestowing the honor, if not self-evident, and the date (e.g., dean's list, 2001)
- *Activities:* the organization or activity and accomplishments
- *Reference phrase:* References available upon request
- *Certificates and licenses:* the name of the license or certificate, licensing agency or organization, and date issued. License numbers are *not* to be included. (License numbers with the name make for easy fraudulent use. When you are actually considered for employment, the employer will ask to see your license so it can be checked with the state board of nursing.)
- *Professional memberships:* the name of the organization, dates of membership, offices held, and special activities
- *Special skills:* for example, languages, computer charting

Format

The next step in creating a résumé is to select a format. The three most common résumé formats are chronological, functional, and a combination of the two. The three formats contain the same basic information about you but are organized in different ways. Your background and job objective will determine the format you use.

The chronological format highlights work experience and education (Figure 3-3). It arranges your work experience in order by dates of the jobs you have had. The most recent job is usually listed first. The functional format is organized around your work experience and the skills involved. For example, you may have provided respite care for your aunt, who has sole responsibility for her invalid mother. In addition, you may have done volunteer work providing respite care for a local hospice, or you may have provided frequent care to your nephew with Down syndrome. These activities could all be listed under one heading that captures the skill of respite care (Figure 3-4). The résumé style that combines both the chronological and functional format is referred to as the combination format (Figure 3-5). The combination format is the one most commonly used for health care résumés. Additional résumé samples are found in Appendix A.

Numerous references are available to help you write a résumé. Tips on effective action words, examples of complete résumés, layout options, and other advice on résumé writing can help you create a high-quality résumé. Ask a friend, a teacher, a coworker, a classmate, or someone else to give you feedback on your résumé. Even after you have revised your résumé 10 times, you will be amazed at the degree to which you can still refine it.

The appearance of your résumé is as important as the content. After all, your résumé may provide employers with their first impression of you. Use direct language. Verbs are to be in the past tense. The résumé should be concise enough to

Anita Jones

1234 Pleasant Street
Chicago, IL 60000
Telephone: (123) 456-7890

OBJECTIVE: Position as an LPN in long-term care setting

LICENSE: Practical Nurse, Illinois Department of Professional Regulation, Issued June 2001

CERTIFICATE: Certified Nursing Assistant (CNA), Illinois Department of Health, Issued May 1998

Certified in CPR, American Red Cross, Issued April 2001

PROFESSIONAL EXPERIENCE:

1998–Present   **General Hospital and Medical Center, Chicago, Illinois**

Position: Certified Nursing Assistant
Provide personal care as a team member on a 38-bed unit

1996–1998   **Heartland Nursing Center, Freeport, Illinois**
Position: Volunteer activity helper

EDUCATION: **Highland Community College, Freeport, Illinois**
Practical Nurse, May 2001

Student representative to hospital committee establishing new procedures and protocols for medication administration

Highland Community College, Freeport, Illinois
Certified Nursing Assistant, June 1998

REFERENCES: Available on request

Figure 3-3 Sample Chronological Résumé

Wong Wu

2686 West Layer
Bismarck, ND 58501
(701) 255-3100

LICENSE:

Registered Nurse, North Dakota Board of Nursing, July 2001

Seeking RN position utilizing the following experience:

- graduating and working as a nurse in Taiwan
- working in the community blood bank while going to school in Bismarck
- graduating from Bismarck Community College, Registered Nurse Program

---

Taiwan

Provided care to surgical patients

Administered medications and IVs as ordered

Blood Bank

Interviewed potential donors

Obtained vital signs

Performed venipuncture to obtain the blood

Bismarck Community College

Volunteered to perform BP screening at senior citizen center

EDUCATION:

University of North Dakota, Bismarck, North Dakota
Currently enrolled in 6 hours of BSN prerequisites

Bismarck Community College, Bismarck, North Dakota
Registered Nurse Program, Diploma May 2001

REFERENCES:

Available on request

Figure 3-4 Sample Functional Résumé

Ludmila Keliehor, RN

796 7th Avenue, Los Angeles, CA 92800   (714) 555-0000

Strengths:
- Supervision
- Role model and mentor
- Recognize needs of client and family
- Discharge planning/teaching

Experience: Medical Center of Southern California,
Los Angeles, California

Registered Nurse, Medical-Surgical, Relief Charge Nurse, August 1996 to present

Care for medical-surgical clients with diabetes, cardiac, respiratory, and surgical diagnoses. Assumed charge nurse role for 38-bed unit.

Selected Accomplishments:
- Wrote and presented classes for diabetic clients
- Preceptor/mentor for new graduates
- Hospital creativity award, 1999, for diabetic classes
- Committees: Quality Assurance

Prior Experience, 1986–1996:

Staff nurse advancing to charge nurse in 26-bed short-stay surgical unit, staff nurse in adult medical-surgical unit

Education: *Associate Degree in Nursing*, 1986, Southern California Community College, Los Angeles, California

Other Professional Education:

Critical care course

Yearly conferences on diabetes care

References: Available on request

Figure 3-5 Sample Combination Résumé

fit on one page. Four pages should be the upper limit. In addition to your qualifications and experiences, what you include on your résumé can be determined by other factors such as the requirements of the job and the interests and pet peeves of the interviewer (recruiter, personnel manager) if you know them (Noble, 2000). The résumé must be typed in a neat, readable typeface (e.g., Times Roman). Your final résumé must be absolutely free of typographical or grammatical errors, erasures, grease smudges, and fingerprints. Good-quality résumé paper should be used: White paper is preferred, although ivory can also be used. Avoid using pastel papers and fancy script typefaces. In addition, avoid logos of any kind. You want to convey competence through a résumé that is professional looking and easy to read.

PREPARE A COVER LETTER

You should prepare a **cover letter**, a letter to accompany a résumé that introduces you and your résumé for the purpose of getting a potential employer's attention. Attach a cover letter to your résumé that is tailored for a specific position. The letter should be one page long, refer to the position you are applying for, explain the way you found out about the position, and briefly describe one of your skills that is pertinent to the position. You should also establish a time frame for contacting the prospective employer to follow up on your résumé. Be sure that you do follow up with a call to track the progress of your application. The letter should follow the standard format of a business letter, contain no grammatical or spelling errors, and be on the same quality paper as your résumé. Always use the full name and title of the person to whom you are sending the letter and résumé. You should not use a stock cover letter for all of the positions for which you are applying. The cover letter should always be individualized to the position and the company to which you are applying. Figure 3-6 shows a sample cover letter.

PREPARE A LIST OF REFERENCES

References are people, such as colleagues, instructors, or employers, who can verify and support your professional and educational background claims.

Through the use of references, prospective employers attempt to verify information you have provided on a job application or your résumé. Employers also use references to gather more information about you. Do not provide references unless the prospective employer requests them. If you must supply references, be sure the list is typed and includes all pertinent information (name, title, employer, address, and telephone number).

Given the likelihood that a potential employer will ask for references, it is a good idea to always be prepared to provide them. Contact the people you intend to list as references and ask whether they are willing to be references for you. Remember, however, that the willingness of a person to serve as a reference does not guarantee that the information provided will be positive; therefore, ask any prospective references how they may respond to questions that you anticipate from a prospective employer. For example, if the employer asks your nursing school instructor

1234 Pleasant Street
Chicago, IL 60000
June 12, 2001

Thomas DiNapoli
Human Resources Manager
St. Anne's Medical Center
P.O. Box 9876
Pittsburgh, PA 15230

Dear Mr. DiNapoli:

I am applying for the position of full-time medication nurse that you advertised in the June 11 *Pittsburgh Press and Post Gazette*. My résumé is enclosed.

In the last year, as student representative, I worked with the hospital committee to establish new procedures and protocols for medication rounds. The procedures have been successfully implemented, and I can bring these innovative ideas to your facility.

I would be happy to come in for an interview. I can be reached at (123) 456-7890 and will call you next week to answer any questions you may have.

Sincerely,

Anita Jones, LPN

Enclosure

Figure 3-6 Sample Cover Letter

something about your record of tardiness, will the instructor focus on the three times you were late for clinical, or will the instructor comment favorably that you are prompt and efficient in completing your responsibilities?

Choose references who are prepared to comment on the skills you possess and need for the job in question. Provide all references with information about the position for which you applied and the job expectations. This information allows your references to tailor their comments to the demands of the prospective job.

PREPARE A TELEPHONE CALL SCRIPT

A telephone call script outlines the information you want to learn or share with prospective employers. Preplanning the telephone call helps you organize the call, ensures that crucial information is learned or given, and generally helps you sound efficient and competent. Consider having several scripts. One script may address a request for information such as job descriptions and vacancies; another may be an introduction about you and an inquiry about the application process; and yet another may focus on the status of your application after you have had an interview. The key is to prepare for any contact with a potential employer, whether it be by phone or in person.

COMPLETE A JOB APPLICATION

Many employers will simply ask you to complete a job application. The job application should be completed totally and neatly. Most employers balk at job applications that say "see attached résumé" rather than provide the information as requested. Preparation is key. Come with the information you may need to complete an application. Such information typically includes a list of past employers, including addresses, telephone numbers, supervisors' names, and dates of employment. Information about schools you have attended is also generally asked for on a job application. If you are nervous about completing an application "cold," ask the employer to send you a form. Practice completing it at home so that you are certain you have all the information requested; then throw the practice application in the trash, and visit the employer to complete the form in person. Figure 3-7 shows a sample job application.

PREPARE FOR THE INTERVIEW

The interview is a crucial part of the job-search process. An interview is best thought of as an opportunity for you and the interviewer to exchange information. Your task is to convey pertinent information about your skills, abilities, education, and experience. The interviewer's task is to relay information about the particular job and the employer and to evaluate your qualifications. If both parties have fulfilled their responsibilities, appropriate decisions follow. The interviewer decides whether you are the most desirable candidate for the job—and you decide whether you want the job.

Preparation is the key to a successful interview. Well before the actual interview, the stage for a meeting is set. You have determined your objective, identified a potential employer, and filled out a job application or provided a résumé. The prospective employer has screened your information and selected you for an interview. But you still have work to do before the actual interview.

Research the Employer

Part of preparing for an interview involves researching the employer. You want to learn everything you can about the employer. Showing such initiative gives the interviewer the impression that you have a sincere interest in employment with the organization. Information you learn may also help you develop questions to ask the employer or anticipate questions that the employer may ask you.

Anticipate Questions

Try to anticipate questions the employer may ask you. For example, if, after investigating an outpatient clinic, you learn that electrocardiogram and phlebotomy are performed on site, you can be fairly certain that the employer will ask whether you have performed these skills. Typical questions asked by an employer focus on strengths and weaknesses, interest in the position, past experience, future plans, and potential contributions to the open position.

Application for Employment
(pre-employment questionnaire) (an equal opportunity employer)

Personal Information

Date _____ June 20, 2001 _____

Name ___ Anita Jones ___

Social security
number ___ 987-65-4321 ___

Present address ___ 1234 Pleasant Street ___ Chicago ___ IL ___ 60000 ___

Permanent address ___ same ___

Phone No. ___ (123) 456-7890 ___   Are you 18 years or older? yes X no

Are you either a U.S. citizen or an alien authorized to work in the United States? yes X no

Employment Desired

Position ___ medication nurse ___ Date you can start ___ October 15 ___ Salary desired ___ open ___

Are you employed now? ___ Yes ___ If so may we inquire of your present employer? ___ Yes ___

Ever applied to this company before? ___ No ___ where? _____ when? _____

Referred by ___ Ken Jenkins ___

Education	Name and location of school attended	No. of years	Did you graduate?	Subjects studied
Grammar school	*Cambden Elementary School District #95*	*8*	*yes*	*general curriculum*
High school	*Cambden High School*	*4*	*yes*	*vocational curriculum, nursing*
College	*Highland Community College*	*1*	*yes*	*LPN*
Trade, business or correspondence school	*Highland Community College*	*6 mo.*	*yes*	*CNA*

Former Employers (list below the last three employers, starting with the last one first)

Date, month and year	Name and address of employer	Salary	Position	Reason for leaving
from 1998 to present	*General Hospital and Medical Center*	*5.90 hr.*	*CNA*	*currently employed*
from to				

Which of these jobs did you like best? _____
What did you like most about this job? ___ *geriatrics* ___

References: give the names of the three persons not related to you, whom you have known at
least one year

Name			
Denise Thompson		friend	10
Phylis Hunter	General Hospital and Medical Center	head nurse	2.5
Frank Hopkins	Highland Community College - Freeport, IL	nursing instructor	1

Figure 3-7 Sample Job Application

As a general rule, law forbids the employer to ask personal questions. For instance, questions about child care arrangements, plans to have a family, height, weight, and religion are not allowed. With severe limitations, the employer can ask about age (e.g., "Are you over 18 or under 70?") and disabilities or illnesses (e.g., "Is there anything that would interfere with your performance of the job?").

Be Prepared

Anticipate questions and plan your responses. Examine your résumé again. Reflect on your goals. Assess your skills and knowledge. Decide what information you want to convey to the interviewer. Develop complete but concise answers to anticipated questions. Employers have a limited amount of time for interviews and want you to get to the point as quickly as possible.

Bring your résumé and references, even if you have already provided them. You want to be certain the interviewer has information about you at hand as you talk.

Be prompt for the interview. An overly early arrival will tend to increase your nervousness; a late arrival is simply unacceptable. Plan your route to the facility ahead of time. Anticipate traffic delays or parking problems. Allow time to compose yourself before the interview.

During the interview you want to make a positive impression. Your physical appearance is probably the first thing the interviewer will notice. Dress conservatively and neatly. You want to project confidence and competence. Excessive jewelry or makeup, trendy body piercing or hairstyle, casual or dirty attire, and overdressing tend to detract from the image you want to present. Examples of professional, conservative dress for a female include a solid-color suit or pantsuit and shoes having flat or small heels. A simple dress is also appropriate. For a male, a solid-color suit with shirt and tie and leather dress shoes or dress pants and sport coat may be worn. Jeans, shorts, T-shirts, sandals, and athletic shoes are not appropriate.

Attempt to present a balanced demeanor: friendly but not too familiar, professional but not too aloof. Greet the interviewer by shaking hands, and wait for the interviewer to offer you a seat. Do not smoke or chew gum. Answer questions directly and honestly, but do not ramble on or offer extraneous information (Figure 3-8).

A common tendency is to view the interview as a one-sided interaction—as the employer's opportunity to scrutinize prospective employees. The interviewer's task is to confirm the information you have provided on your job application or résumé. In addition to gathering more detailed information about you, the interviewer is interested in the way you handle yourself and whether you are a good match for the job and the employer. After a screening and selection process, the employer offers employment to the most desirable candidate. But remember, securing employment is a two-sided process: You also are interviewing the interviewer to gather information about the employer, to ascertain whether the job opportunity is the right fit for you.

Any offer of employment you receive can be accepted or rejected. You should already have obtained information about the employer that was enticing enough to cause you to apply for employment. The interview is, however, your opportunity

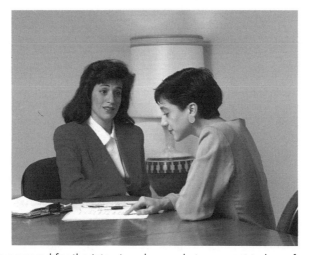

Figure 3-8 Be prepared for the interview; know what you want to learn from and what you want to share with the interviewer.

to gather more information about the employer. This information serves as the basis for determining whether you really want the job. Go to the interview with a written list of questions you have for the employer.

Your questions can address a number of topics, including orientation, organization of the nursing staff, working conditions, and educational opportunities. For example: How long is the orientation? How often is overtime or floating required? On which unit will I be assigned to work? What are the five most common diagnoses on that unit? What is the ratio of RNs to LP/VNs to UAP? What is the schedule of a normal work week? The list of potential questions is endless.

The advice is often given not to ask about salary and benefits during the first interview. At some point, however, this information becomes crucial to your decision making. If the interviewer does not volunteer information about salary and benefits, at the very least wait until the end of the interview to discuss these matters. Employers want to know you are interested in the work, not just the pay. Thus, you may want to consider waiting to learn about salary and benefits until a job offer has been made.

At the end of the interview, you may be offered employment. If you are confident that you want the position, accept the offer. If you have any hesitation, however, inform the employer that you will respond in a day or two. Do not turn the offer down at the interview. Go home, review the information you have available, discuss the offer with relevant people, and then notify the employer. Whether you decide to accept or decline the offer of employment, you should respond to the employer's offer. Even in declining an employment offer, you want to leave a positive impression. You never know when you may encounter that recruiter in the future.

At the end of the interview, shake hands with the interviewer and offer thanks for the interviewer's time and consideration. If you believe you want the job, say so. Statements such as "After our discussion, I am very interested in working here" or "I really want to work with your client population" indicate your strong interest to the prospective employer.

PREPARE A THANK YOU NOTE

The thank you note is critical to a successful job search. Always follow up an interview with a thank you note. Some employment counselors suggest you send a thank you note to everyone involved in the interview process. These people may include the person who suggested the employer, the receptionist, and, certainly, the person who conducted the interview.

A thank you note can be handwritten or typed. The key is to send it the same day as the interview. The thank you note should be personal: Say something about the way the person treated you, the highlights of the interview, or something you forgot to mention during the interview. If the interview confirmed your interest in employment, say so. Even if you decide that the employment setting is not for you, write a thank you note. Your career interests may change at some point. Further, employers talk to each other; therefore, you want to leave a good impression any place you seek employment. Figure 3-9 shows a sample thank you note.

1234 Pleasant Street
Chicago, IL 60000
June 26, 2001

Thomas DiNapoli
Human Resources Manager
St. Anne's Medical Center
P.O. Box 9876
Pittsburgh, PA 15230

Dear Mr. DiNapoli:

Thank you for taking the time to speak with me today about the position of medication nurse at St. Anne's Medical Center. I was very impressed with your company, and the job sounds wonderful. I'm more than ever convinced that my experience can benefit your company.

I appreciated the opportunity to meet you and learn about St. Anne's.

Sincerely,

Anita Jones, LPN

Figure 3-9 Sample Thank You Note

A FINAL WORD ABOUT EMPLOYMENT

As a new graduate, you may find that your job search is influenced by financial pressures or a seemingly limited pool of available jobs. You also may be considerably swayed by the advice that you should "get a year of experience in general medical-surgical nursing" before moving on to the job you really want. Financial pressures and the job market may indeed pose some limitations. Further, a year of medical-surgical experience is helpful. But resist taking a job for just these reasons.

As an occupation, nursing offers much variety with regard to employment setting, client age, type of work, number of hours available to work, availability of days and shifts, amount of supervision, and a host of other factors. Such variety will become evident as you investigate available employment options.

A poor fit between the job and your interests, needs, or abilities is a setup for failure. As a newly employed nurse, you want to establish an employment record of success and increasing growth in your skills and knowledge. You want to build on your newfound confidence and competence. A thorough and honest evaluation of your strengths and weaknesses, a clearly identified objective, and a careful review of employment options will help ensure satisfying and rewarding employment.

SUMMARY

- The steps involved in securing a job include identifying your objective, preparing a résumé, preparing a cover letter, preparing a list of references, preparing a telephone call script, completing a job application, preparing for the interview, and preparing a thank you note.
- The format of a résumé may be chronological, functional, or a combination of the two.
- Contact the persons you intend to list as references and ask whether they are willing to provide a reference for you. Ask how they may respond to questions that you anticipate from a prospective employer.
- Prepare for the interview by doing research about the employer and by thinking about the questions the employer may ask.
- For the interview, dress conservatively and neatly; be clean; be prompt; bring your résumé and references; wait for the interviewer to offer you a seat; do not smoke or chew gum.
- Always follow up an interview with a thank you note, sent on the same day as the interview.

Review Questions

1. The following information should be included on a résumé:
    a. Name, address, telephone number, job objective
    b. Information about previous employment, name, family information
    c. Job objective, references, education, work experiences
    d. Name, address, job objective, availability for interview

2. The persons you provide as references should be able to:

   a. verify your membership in professional organizations.
   b. verify and support your professional and educational claims.
   c. answer questions about what you have done during your life.
   d. meet with the prospective employer for a discussion about you.

3. Send a cover letter:

   a. with the résumé.
   b. when declining a job offer.
   c. when accepting a job offer.
   d. to inquire about a job opening.

Critical Thinking Questions

1. After a lengthy job search, Alicia secures employment at a long-term care facility. The facility residents are all retired nuns. Alicia enjoys geriatrics; management seemed fair and reasonable; the environment is clean and attractive; and financial benefits are competitive. However, Alicia finds the nuns to be demanding and unappreciative. In addition, the religious underpinnings of the facility influence her work more than she anticipated. After 2 months, she now dreads going to work. What should she do?

2. Compare the chronological résumé at the right with the one in Figure 3-3. Which one is better? Why?

WEB FLASH!

- Search the Web under broad categories such as *job hunting*, *seeking jobs*, or *finding jobs*. What kind of sites do you locate?
- Now search for *résumés*, *cover letters*, and *interviewing*. Are the sites the same as for above? Which sites are most helpful?
- Check the major search engines such as www.yahoo.com and www.altavista.com for jobs, résumés, and so on.

References/Suggested Readings

Bolles, R. N. (2000). *What color is your parachute? A practical manual for job-hunters & career-changers.* Berkeley, CA: Ten Speed Press.
Case, B. (1997). *Career planning for nurses.* Albany, NY: Delmar.
Diggs, A. D. (1999). *Barrier-breaking resumes & interviews.* New York: Times Books.
Haft, T. (1997). *Job notes: Resumes.* New York: Princeton Review Publishing, L.L.C.

Anita Jones
1234 Pleasant Street
Chicago, IL 60000
Telephone: (123) 456-7890

OBJECTIVE: Position as an LPN in long-term care setting

LICENSE NUMBER: State of Illinois # _____

PROFESSIONAL EXPERIENCE:

1992–Present
**General Hospital and Medical Center
Chicago, Illinois**

Position: LPN, medication nurse

Provide direct care as a team member on a 38-bed unit. Distribute and maintain medications. Work in cooperation with nonlicensed team members. Manage nursing outcomes using assistive personnel. Received three letters of commendation for patient care delivery.

1987–1992
**City Teaching Medical Center
Chicago, Illinois**

Position: LPN, general medical unit

Provided direct patient care on a 25-bed unit. Gained experience caring for geriatric patients. Helped develop unit procedures for shift rotation. Participated in an average of 12 hours of continuing-education contact hours per year.

EDUCATION:
Chicago State University, Chicago, Illinois

Completed 24 credit hours of course work in BSN prerequisites, focus on physiology and psychology

Highland Community College, Freeport, Illinois

Licensed Practical Nurse, 1987

Class representative to faculty council

RELATED EXPERIENCE:
Lectured 25 preschool students on keeping healthy, repeated program four times

AFFILIATIONS: Member, NFLPN

REFERENCES: Available upon request

Kay, A. (1997). *Resumes that will get you the job you want*. Cincinnati, OH: Betterway Books.

Krannich, C., & Krannich, R. (1998). *Interview for success: A practical guide to increasing job interviews, offers, and salaries* (7th ed.). Manassas Park, VA: Impact Publications.

Marino, K. (1997). *Just resumes: 200 powerful and proven successful resumes to get that job* (2nd ed.). New York: John Wiley & Sons.

Marino, K. (2000). *Resumes for the health care professional* (2nd ed.). New York: John Wiley & Sons.

Martin, E., & Langhorne, K. (1995). *Cover letters they don't forget*. Lincolnwood, IL: VGM Career Horizons.

Mattera, M. D. (Ed.). (1997). Ace the all-important job interview. In *Nursing opportunities 1997*. Montvale, NJ: Medical Economics.

Noble, D. (2000). *Gallery of best resumes* (2nd ed.). Indianapolis, IN: JIST Works.

Parker, Y. (1996). *Damn good resume guide: A crash course in resume writing* (3rd ed.). Berkeley, CA: Ten Speed Press.

Pontow, R. (1999). *Proven resumes: Strategies that have increased salaries and changed lives*. Berkeley, CA: Ten Speed Press.

Smith, R. (2000). *Electronic resumes & online networking*. Franklin Lakes, NJ: Career Press.

VGM's Professional Resumes Series. (1999). *Resumes for scientific and technical careers* (2nd ed.). Lincolnwood, IL: VGM Career Horizons.

WORKPLACE TRANSITION

CHAPTER 4

LEARNING OBJECTIVES

Upon completion of this chapter, you should be able to:
- *Define key terms.*
- *Describe the roles, level of education, skills, level of independence, and length of education for the various members of the nursing staff.*
- *Compare and contrast policies and procedures.*
- *Explain an organizational chart.*

KEY TERMS

competencies	evaluation	policies
conflict	job description	procedures
confrontation	organizational chart	

INTRODUCTION

A successful employment experience depends on more than nursing knowledge and technical competence. Success requires competence in the particular job position. Success also depends on the nurse's integration into the health care team and the nurse's understanding of the overall health care organization.

THE NURSING TEAM

Within the nursing staff are different team members. Nursing staff includes nursing UAP, CNAs, LP/VNs, RNs, and nurse practitioners (NPs). The roles, levels of education, skills, levels of independence, and lengths of education vary considerably (Figure 4-1). Familiarizing yourself with the roles of other nursing staff will help ensure that your practice conforms to the scope of practice as outlined by law.

In nursing, a UAP can have a number of different titles, including UAP, patient care technician, clinical technician, and nursing assistant. These persons provide

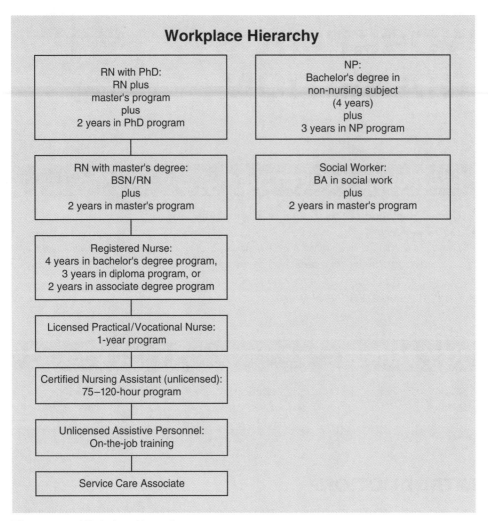

Figure 4-1 Workplace Hierarchy

![step icon] **PROFESSIONAL TIP**

Unlicensed Personnel

Much controversy surrounds the role of UAP. Concerns have been raised that unlicensed personnel are functioning as de facto licensed nurses in violation of Nursing Practice Acts. Further, serious questions exist about the cost savings and quality of care in light of increased reliance on UAP and a corresponding reduction in licensed nurses. Understanding the role and limitations of UAP is critical.

Hierarchy

As defined in the Nursing Practice Acts, or in the state nursing board's rules and regulations, an LP/VN works under the direction of an RN, physician, or dentist. These are the professionals who will directly supervise your work. In some states, the language of the law indicates that "other health care providers" can supervise you. The question is, Who are the other health care providers? In your state, must you follow orders written by a physician's assistant? A nurse practitioner? A physical therapist? The answers vary by state. It is critical that you know who can direct your nursing activities.

hands-on care to clients in addition to performing other duties. None of these personnel has a license to practice. Rather, training is provided by the employer and may last from 2 to 10 weeks. The tasks they are expected to perform are designated by the employer and typically include things such as phlebotomy, electrocardiogram measurement, intake and output reading, bed making, and assisting clients with activities of daily living.

A CNA is also unlicensed. In contrast to those for other UAP, however, the curriculum and length of training to become a CNA are prescribed. As part of health care reforms in the long-term care setting, the primary employment setting of CNAs, a set curriculum of 100 hours' duration must be completed to be certified.

Licensed practical/vocational nurses work very closely with registered nurses. The LP/VN attends a 1-year program and must pass the National Council Licensure Examination for Practical Nurses (NCLEX-PN®). The RN is educated in a 3-year hospital-diploma program, a 2-year college associate-degree program, or a 4-year college baccalaureate program and must pass the National Council Licensure Examination for Registered Nurses (NCLEX-RN®).

An NP is an RN who has obtained additional education (usually a master's degree) and is certified by the state. The role of the NP typically includes diagnosis and treatment of commonly occurring medical conditions. Outpatient clinics frequently employ NPs. Increasingly, they are also found working in hospitals, long-term care facilities, and rehabilitation centers.

JOB EXPECTATIONS AND RESPONSIBILITIES

Employees are hired to work at a specific site, for example, the fifth floor of the hospital or the internal medicine clinic at the outpatient health facility. The employer's expectations are summarized in job descriptions and in the policy and procedure manual. Although reading these papers is often viewed as boring and a waste of time, successful employment depends on understanding job expectations and the employer's policies.

Job Descriptions

A **job description** is a written outline of job responsibilities. Job responsibilities vary from employer to employer. For example, in long-term care facilities, LP/VNs are not routinely expected to bathe clients, as this task is performed by CNAs. In a hospital setting, however, job responsibilities of an LP/VN or RN may include bathing clients. All the job expectations should fall within the scope of practice of the nurse.

In addition to summarizing job responsibilities, a job description frequently outlines requirements for the position (e.g., LP/VN, experience preferred), supervisor's title, supervisory responsibilities, and frequency and method of evaluation. A job description may also include a list of **competencies**, the specific skills or tasks (e.g., blood glucose monitoring) needed for a particular position. Employers are expected to assess competencies at the time of employment and periodically thereafter, usually annually.

A clear understanding of one's own job description is critical to the safe, effective practice of nursing in the specific employment setting. Failure to meet the job responsibilities as outlined in the job description can result in termination of employment. Familiarity with the job descriptions of supervisors and of persons who you may supervise is also very helpful in ensuring that you have a clear understanding of your role and what you can expect of others.

Policies and Procedures

The employer's policies and procedure manual is also a very important reference document.

An employer's **policies** are written descriptions of the employer's expectations for handling various situations. Policies often are applicable to everyone working in the facility, rather than being nursing specific. Policies addressing confidentiality, dissemination of client information, handling of suspected cases of abuse, management of client valuables, and so on are common. A review of the policies and procedures manual is often required at the start of employment. A periodic self-initiated review of the manual is useful in ensuring that work performance meets the employer's expectations.

Procedures are step-by-step instructions describing the processes for performing various nursing tasks. Although these nursing procedures will likely be familiar to you, it is important that you perform tasks as directed by your employer. There are usually several correct, safe methods for performing a procedure; the way you were taught in school may vary from your employer's procedure. This difference may require altering the way you perform certain procedures

Evaluation

Evaluation, the act of examining and judging the quality and degree to which a person performs the expected duties, is very familiar to new nursing graduates. During the nursing program, instructors frequently evaluate each student. Once you have become an employed nurse, evaluations will continue. Now, however, the criteria for evaluation will be your job description and the agency's policies and procedures rather than course and clinical objectives.

Job Evaluation

Constructive evaluation is directed toward the person's behavior and has no bearing on the person's value. Although new graduates are seldom, if ever, responsible for formally evaluating others, a new graduate may decide to give feedback (another word for evaluation) to a coworker regarding specific behavior observed. It is important to be sensitive to personality differences between you and the person receiving the feedback. Feedback should be given privately, soon after the behavior is observed. Try to begin with something positive and then focus on what could be improved. Listen actively to the other person to avoid misunderstandings. On occasion, give only positive feedback.

When you are the recipient of feedback, try to remain objective. The feedback is about your behavior, not about your value as a person. If the feedback is about some way in which you need to improve in carrying out your professional responsibilities, think if you have heard the same feedback from anyone else. If you have, the feedback probably has some merit. Acknowledge the feedback; plan how you can do things differently; then carry out your plan. Above all, do not make excuses and do not react defensively. Try to see the benefits of the feedback.

Self-Evaluation

As you begin your career, and throughout your work life, it is beneficial to evaluate yourself. At the end of each day, take a few minutes to think about your behaviors in carrying out your duties. Did you always perform procedures safely? Did you perform the procedures according to the procedure manual, or did you take shortcuts that may have adversely affected the client? Were you courteous to your coworkers and helpful to others?

At the end of the day, list one or two professional traits that you intend to improve on the next day. Each day, look at the list as you evaluate yourself. On some days you may add to the list; on others, you may mark off some items.

Do not be afraid to ask for help from an experienced nurse. Discussing your duties with an experienced nurse often provides a wealth of information that is helpful in providing quality care to your clients.

Conflict and Confrontation

Most persons hope for situations in which everyone gets along and all goes smoothly. However, conflict is a normal aspect of relationships. **Conflict**, a clash, competition, or mutual interference of opposing forces or qualities (e.g., ideas, interests), can be severe (sharp disagreement or fighting) or mild (subtle or unconscious opposition to an idea or action). Conflict is often thought about negatively. Thinking critically about conflict provides an opportunity to achieve realistic outcomes and to gain personal growth.

It is wise to be aware of your natural style of dealing with conflict. Five styles used in managing conflict have been identified (Alfaro-LeFevre, 1999):

- *Avoiders* ignore the situation or persons believed to be causing the conflict. Problems are allowed to continue.
- *Accommodators* try to make others feel better. They may explode when things get too bad.
- *Forcers* work to have their way. They are indifferent about whether they are liked.
- *Compromisers* try to persuade everyone to give a little. Their solutions generally are minimally acceptable, and conflict often continues.
- *Collaborative problem solvers* work to face issues together. They address both the situation and relationships involved. They seek solutions by finding areas of agreement and differences, evaluating alternatives, and choosing solutions supported by all parties involved.

When conflict occurs, many people criticize, betray confidences, or gossip. It takes courage to confront a situation or person. **Confrontation** is the act of facing an unpleasant situation or a person who has opposing views. The person who deals with confrontation in an honest, open, and kind manner is trusted and respected.

ORGANIZATIONAL CHART

An **organizational chart** is a visual representation of the relationships of one department to another within the facility or the relationship of the facility to other facilities in a health care network. Included in the organizational chart are the titles of department leaders and the lines of authority. This information provides an understanding of the way a department fits into the larger organization (Figure 4-2).

All employees within a health care facility are part of a large organization. Every organization has a unique organizational culture of commonly held values, beliefs, and expectations directing the work force in the provision of services. For example, the organizational culture of a for-profit freestanding kidney dialysis center will be different from that of a free health clinic. Insights into the organizational culture of any health care facility can be garnered from the organization statement summarizing the facility's mission, vision, values, and goals. Although such statements often seem theoretical and far removed from job responsibilities, they do guide the organization in its provision of services.

SUMMARY

- The nursing team includes nurse practitioners (NPs), registered nurses (RNs), licensed practical/vocational nurses (LP/VNs), certified nursing assistants (CNAs), and unlicensed assistive personnel (UAP).
- A job description is a written outline of job responsibilities.
- An organization's policies are written descriptions of the employer's expectations for handling various situations.
- Procedures are step-by-step instructions for performing various nursing tasks.

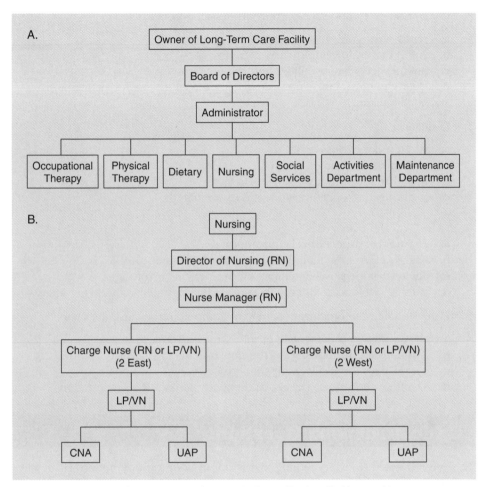

Figure 4-2 Sample Organizational Charts: A. Entire Facility; B. Nursing Unit

- Conflict can be a growth-producing experience.
- The organizational chart shows the relationship of one department to another within a facility and the relationships within a department.

Review Questions

1. The LP/VN may supervise:

   a. two-year RNs.
   b. only other LP/VNs.
   c. only CNAs and UAP.
   d. other LP/VNs, CNAs, and UAP.

2. It is important to understand your job description because it:

    a. states what you can and cannot do.
    b. is the reason for employment termination.
    c. outlines job responsibilities and requirements.
    d. clearly outlines instructions describing the processes for performing nursing care.

3. Evaluation:

    a. is often done in groups.
    b. always has the same criteria.
    c. is directed toward a person's behavior.
    d. is not needed once the student has graduated.

4. Conflict:

    a. is a normal aspect of relationships.
    b. has no place in nursing because it disrupts client care.
    c. always has negative outcomes on the persons involved.
    d. is to be avoided at all costs because some people become very angry.

5. Understanding the organizational chart is important because the chart:

    a. shows how you personally fit into the organization.
    b. diagrams the relationship of the departments in a facility.
    c. summarizes the facility's mission, vision, values, and goals.
    d. identifies the values, beliefs, and expectations of the organization.

Critical Thinking Questions

1. You are asked to do something that is not in your job description. How will you handle the situation?

2. How often should you read the policies of the facility where you are working?

WEB FLASH!

- Search the Web for the home page of the facility where you are working. Does it have one? What information is available there? How is this information valuable to you?

Reference

Alfaro-LeFevre, R. (1999). *Critical thinking in nursing: A practical approach*. Philadelphia: Saunders.

Sample Résumés

CHRONOLOGICAL RÉSUMÉ

Andra Visosky
6754 West Seventh Street
Oak Park, IL 60430
(630) 904-8208

CAREER OBJECTIVE To obtain a Licensed Practical Nurse position with a hospital or long-term care facility

EDUCATION College of DuPage, Lombard, Illinois

Licensed Practical Nursing Program, Certificate, 2001

GPA 3.8/4.0, Dean's List

Member: Phi Theta Kappa, National Honor Society

Triton College, River Grove, Illinois

Nurse Assistant Program, CNA Certificate, 1995

EXPERIENCE

Aug. 2000–Present Sun Home Health Agency, River Forest Illinois
Home Health Aide
Employed part time while in school

May 1998–July 2000 Home Care Plus, Evanston, Illinois
Home Health Aide

Sept. 1997–April 1998 Park Community Hospital, Aurora, Illinois
CNA–Critical Care

Experience Summary Rest Haven Nursing Home, Wheaton, Illinois
1993–1997 **CNA**

South Shore Nursing Home, Blue Island, Illinois
Activity Assistant, Dietary Assistant

REFERENCES Available on request

FUNCTIONAL RÉSUMÉ

James Olivarez
(361) 992-7890

3813 Yorktown Road
Corpus Christi, TX 78400

LICENSE: Vocational Nurse, Texas Board of Vocational Nurse Examiners, June 2001

Seek LP/VN position utilizing the following experience

- Providing respite care monthly for my aunt who cares for my grandmother
- Providing respite care as volunteer through a local hospice
- Graduating recently from Del Mar College, Vocational Nursing Program
- Speaking Spanish fluently

RESPITE CARE

Provided personal hygiene and grooming.

Assisted client in performing range-of-motion exercises.

Prepared meals and assisted client with food intake.

Kept accurate intake and output records.

Toileted client every three hours.

Assisted client to ambulate or sit in chair three times a day.

Administered medications as ordered.

Participated in diversional activities (e.g., playing games, listening to music, reading to client) as suggested by family or requested by client.

EDUCATION: **Del Mar College, Corpus Christi, Texas**, currently enrolled in 6 hours of ADN prerequisites

Del Mar College, Corpus Christi, Texas, Vocational Nurse Program, Certificate, May 2001

REFERENCES: Available on request

COMBINATION RÉSUMÉ

Lyvonne Selvera, RN
1010 Coble Glen Court
Durham, NC 27700
(919) 544-7317

PROFILE

Efficient, caring registered nurse with well-rounded experience attained through increasingly responsible positions in clinical health settings. Skills include direct client care and IV proficiency. Knowledge and skills updated regularly through continuing education workshops. Currently working on gerontological nursing certification.

HIGHLIGHTS OF QUALIFICATIONS

- 8 years of nursing experience
- Recognized by a previous employer for writing client-teaching guides, and complimented by supervisors for concise, quality documentation
- Excellent organizational and time-management skills
- Familiar with policies and adhere to them

PROFESSIONAL EXPERIENCE

1996–Present   Rex Hospital, Durham, North Carolina
Staff Nurse
- Work with 4 other nurses on 36-bed unit.
- Establish appropriate care plans for clients and their families.
- Provide teaching to client and family: diseases, precautions and restrictions, proper medication use, medication side effects, and diet.
- Provide direct client care for cardiac and stroke clients; care includes performing physical and disease process assessments, administering medications including IV therapy, performing cardiac monitoring, and changing dressings.
- Precept student nurses and new employees.

(continued)

1992–1996   Durham Community Hospital, Durham, North Carolina

Staff Nurse   (1995–1996)

Licensed Practical Nurse   (1992–1995)

- Performed client care. Taught care to clients and families, including discharge teaching on 24-bed respiratory unit. Assisted physicians with bedside procedures.
- As **Staff Nurse**, filled in as evening charge nurse and accepted the role of resource person for students and orientees.
- Wrote client teaching guide: Use of incentive spirometry.

EDUCATION

Associate Degree in Nursing, Durham Technical College, Durham, North Carolina, 1995

Honors: Dean's list, Graduated cum laude

Practical Nurse Diploma, Durham Technical College, Durham, North Carolina, 1992

CPR certified (current)

Continuing Education

Workshops include respiratory care, gerontology (preparing for certification), wound care, HIV, and AIDS

ACTIVITIES

National Federation of Licensed Practical Nurses (NFLPN), local board member

Volunteer for American Heart Association

COMBINATION RÉSUMÉ

Elmon Hendi

431 Rightway Drive	Telephone/Message
Birmingham, AL 35200	(205) 995-3151

OBJECTIVE   Seeking position as **Licensed Practical Nurse**

OVERVIEW
- Highly motivated new graduate, compassionate, dedicated to quality client care
- Organized and efficient
- Very capable in performing client assessments and client care, administering medications, documentation including computer charting

EDUCATION
- Licensed Practical Nurse, Diploma June 2001, Birmingham Technical College, Birmingham, Alabama, Graduated with **honors**
- Received clinical experience at the following health care facilities:

Webb County Hospital:	Psychiatric unit
Kirby Community Hospital:	OB/GYN & Medical/Surgical
Alabama Children's Hospital:	Pediatrics

EXPERIENCE   **Pharmaceutical Salesman**, 1985–1998

XYZ Company
- Called on physicians at their offices, receiving feedback about medications
- Made presentations to physician organizations regarding new medications

Salesperson, 1998–2001

Part time while in school 2000–2001

ABC Car Parts, Birmingham, Alabama
- Assisted customers in determining correct parts for their make and model of vehicle
- Kept inventory neatly stocked

Received commendation from company for having many customer appreciation letters.

LICENSE   Alabama Board of Nursing, Licensed Practical Nurse, July 2001

REFERENCES   Available on request

COMBINATION RÉSUMÉ

Selina Duperier, LPN
4205 Waite Street
Bellevue, WA 98000
(425) 321-5689

EDUCATION
Bellevue Community College
Practical Nurse Diploma, May 2001

CURRENT CERTIFICATION
CPR 4/01–4/02

EMPLOYMENT HISTORY

5/00–4/01 Picks Grocery, Bellevue, Washington
Cashier—Part time while going to school

8/90–4/00 Smith Elementary School, Seattle, Washington
Secretary—Liaison to parents. Routed telephone calls. Drafted and typed correspondence. Administered first aid. Maintained accurate student records. Performed light bookkeeping.

2/85–8/90 Tourism & Economic Development, Seattle, Washington
Fundraiser—Gave presentations to large and small groups to elicit support for organization-sponsored programs. Helped plan and organize fundraising events.

LICENSE
Washington State Nursing Care Quality Assurance Commission
Licensed Practical Nurse, June 2001

REFERENCES AVAILABLE ON REQUEST

COMBINATION RÉSUMÉ

Akiko Kiona
6558 East Boston Street
Bryan, OH 43500
(419) 746-3191

OBJECTIVE: To obtain a rewarding position as a **Registered Nurse**

HIGHLIGHTS OF QUALIFICATIONS
- Current Licensed Registered Nurse in the State of Ohio
- Genuine concern for clients
- Manage time efficiently and effectively
- Reliable self-starter
- Remain focused under stress

EDUCATION
Associate of Science Degree in Nursing, May 2001
Cleveland Community College, Cleveland, Ohio
GPA 3.7/4.0

High School Diploma, May 2000
Bryan Consolidated School, Bryan, Ohio
GPA 3.8/4.0

SUMMARY OF EXPERIENCE
- Excellent clinical evaluations throughout nursing program
- Drill team captain in high school
- Member of high school debate team; received top state honors

LICENSE/CERTIFICATION
Licensed Registered Nurse, Ohio Board of Nursing, June 2001

CPR certified (current)

References Provided on Request

COMBINATION RÉSUMÉ

Wade Boedeker
10910 Cypress Creek Drive
Roswell, NM 88200
(505) 853-2171

OBJECTIVE:

To gain valuable experience as a **Registered Nurse** in the medical-surgical unit of a major hospital

SUMMARY OF QUALIFICATIONS:

- Received A.D. in Nursing from Santa Fe Community College, May 2001
- Motivated and dedicated to providing professional, quality client care
- Maintain excellent relationships with clients, family, staff, and administration
- Effective time management skills

EDUCATION:

A.D. Nursing—May 2001
Santa Fe Community College—Santa Fe, New Mexico

CPR certified (current)

Scheduled to take NCLEX-RN June 2001

HEALTH CARE EXPERIENCE:

Nurse Technician—June 2000–present
County Hospital—Santa Fe, New Mexico

- Provide client care
- Remove sutures, dress wounds, give injections, and administer other treatments as required

References and Additional Information Available on Request

APPENDIX B

Boards of Nursing

Alabama Board of Nursing; 770 Washington Avenue; RSA Plaza, Suite 250; Montgomery, AL 36130-3900; 334-242-4060; www.abn.state.al.us/

Alaska Board of Nursing; Dept. of Comm. & Econ. Development; Division of Occupational Licensing; 3601 C Street, Suite 722; Anchorage, AK 99503; 907-269-8161; www.dced.state.ak.us/occ/pnur.htm

American Samoa Health Services; Services Regulatory Board; LBJ Tropical Medical Center; Pago Pago, AS 96799; 684-633-1222

Arizona State Board of Nursing; 1651 East Morten Avenue, Suite 210; Phoenix, AZ 85020; 602-331-8111; www.azboardofnursing.org/

Arkansas State Board of Nursing; University Tower Building; 1123 South University, Suite 800; Little Rock, AR 72204-1619; 501-686-2700; www.state.ar.us/nurse

California Board of Registered Nursing; 400 R Street, Suite 4030; Sacramento, CA 95814-6239; 916-322-3350; www.rn.ca.gov/

California Board of Vocational Nurse and Psychiatric Technician Examiners; 2535 Capitol Oaks Drive, Suite 205; Sacramento CA 95833; 916-263-7800; www.bvnpt.ca.gov/

Colorado Board of Nursing; 1560 Broadway, Suite 880; Denver, CO 80202; 303-894-2430; www.dora.state.co.us/nursing/

Connecticut Board of Examiners for Nursing; Department of Public Health; 410 Capitol Avenue, MS# 13PHO; P.O. Box 340308; Hartford, CT 06134-0328; 860-509-7624; www.state.ct.us/dph/

Delaware Board of Nursing; 861 Silver Lake Boulevard; Cannon Building, Suite 203; Dover, DE 19904; 302-739-4522

District of Columbia Board of Nursing; Department of Health; 825 North Capitol Street, N.E., 2nd Floor; Room 2224; Washington, DC 20002; 202-442-4778

Florida Board of Nursing; 4080 Woodcock Drive, Suite 202; Jacksonville, FL 32207; 904-858-6940; www.doh.state.fl.us/mqa/nursing/rnhome.htm

Georgia State Board of Licensed Practical Nurses; 237 Coliseum Drive; Macon, GA 31217-3858; 912-207-1300; www.sos.state.ga.us/ebd-lpn

Georgia Board of Nursing; 237 Coliseum Drive; Macon, GA 31217-3858; 912-207-1660; www.sos.state.ga.us/ebd-rn/

Guam Board of Nurse Examiners; P.O. Box 2816; 1304 East Sunset Boulevard; Barrgada, GU 96913; 671-475-0251

Hawaii Board of Nursing; Professional & Vocational Licensing Division; P.O. Box 3469; Honolulu, HI 96801; 808-586-3000; www.state.hi.us/dcca/pvloffline/

Idaho Board of Nursing; 280 North 8th Street, Suite 210; P.O. Box 83720; Boise, ID 83720; 208-334-3110; www.state.id.us/ibn/ibnhome.htm

Illinois Department of Professional Regulation; James R. Thompson Center; 100 West Randolph, Suite 9-300; Chicago, IL 60601; 312-814-2715; www.dpr.state.il.us/

Indiana State Board of Nursing; Health Professions Bureau; 402 West Washington Street, Room W041; Indianapolis, IN 46204; 317-232-2960; www.state.in.us/hbp/boards/isbn/

Iowa Board of Nursing; RiverPoint Business Park; 400 S.W. 8th Street, Suite B; Des Moines, IA 50309-4685; 515-281-3255; www.state.ia.us/government/nursing/

Kansas State Board of Nursing; Landon State Office Building; 900 S.W. Jackson, Suite 551-S; Topeka, KS 66612; 785-296-4929; www.ksbn.org

Kentucky Board of Nursing; 312 Whittington Parkway, Suite 300; Louisville, KY 40222; 502-329-7000; www.kbn.state.ky.us/

Louisiana State Board of Practical Nurse Examiners; 3421 North Causeway Boulevard, Suite 203; Metairie, LA 70002; 504-838-5791; www.lsbpne.com

Louisiana State Board of Nursing; 3510 North Causeway Boulevard, Suite 501; Metairie, LA 70003; 504-838-5332; www.lsbn.state.la.us/

Maine State Board of Nursing; 158 State House Station; Augusta, ME 04333; 207-287-1133; www.state.me.us/nursingbd/

Maryland Board of Nursing; 4140 Patterson Avenue; Baltimore, MD 21215; 410-585-1900; www.mbon.org

Massachusetts Board of Registration in Nursing; Commonwealth of Massachusetts; 239 Causeway Street; Boston, MA 02114; 617-727-9961; www.state.ma.us/reg/boards/rn/

Michigan CIS/Office of Health Services; Ottawa Towers North; 611 West Ottawa, 4th Floor; Lansing, MI 48933; 517-373-9102; www.cis.state.mi.us/bhser/genover.htm

Minnesota Board of Nursing; 2829 University Avenue SE, Suite 500; Minneapolis, MN 55414; 612-617-2270; www.nursingboard.state.mn.us/

Mississippi Board of Nursing; 1935 Lakeland Drive, Suite B; Jackson, MS 39216-5014; 601-987-4188; www.msbn.state.ms.us/

Missouri State Board of Nursing; 3605 Missouri Boulevard; P.O. Box 656; Jefferson City, MO 65102-0656; 573-751-0681; www.ecodev.state.mo.us/pr/nursing/

Montana State Board of Nursing; 301 South Park; Helena, MT 59620-0513; 406-444-2071; www.com.state.mt.us/License/POL/index.htm

Commonwealth Board of Nurse Examiners; Capitol Hill; Building 1336; Saipan, MP 96950; 670-664-4810

Nebraska Health and Human Services System; Department of Regulation & Licensure, Nursing Section; 301 Centennial Mall South; Lincoln, NE 68509-4986; 402-471-4376; www.hhs.state.ne.us/crl/nns.htm

Nevada State Board of Nursing; 1755 East Plumb Lane, Suite 260; Reno, NV 89502; 775-688-2620; www.nursingboard.state.nv.us

New Hampshire Board of Nursing; P.O. Box 3898; 78 Regional Drive, BLDG B; Concord, NH 03302; 603-271-2323; www.state.nh.us/nursing/

New Jersey Board of Nursing; P.O. Box 45010; 124 Halsey Street, 6th Floor; Newark, NJ 07101; 973-504-6586; www.state.nj.us/lps/ca/medical.htm

New Mexico Board of Nursing; 4206 Louisiana Boulevard, NE; Suite A; Albuquerque, NM 87109; 505-841-8340; www.state.nm.us/clients/nursing

New York State Board of Nursing; Education Building; 89 Washington Avenue; 2nd Floor West Wing; Albany, NY 12234; 518-474-3817; www.nysed.gov/prof/nurse.htm

North Carolina Board of Nursing; 3724 National Drive, Suite 201; Raleigh NC 27612; 919-782-3211; www.ncbon.com/

North Dakota Board of Nursing; 919 South 7th Street, Suite 504; Bismarck, ND 58504; 701-328-9777; www.ndbon.org/

Ohio Board of Nursing; 17 South High Street, Suite 400; Columbus, OH 43215-3413; 614-466-3947; www.state.oh.us/nur/

Oklahoma Board of Nursing; 2915 North Classen Boulevard, Suite 524; Oklahoma City, OK 73106; 405-962-1800

Oregon State Board of Nursing; 800 NE Oregon Street, Box 25; Suite 465; Portland, OR 97232; 503-731-4745; www.osbn.state.or.us/

Pennsylvania State Board of Nursing; 124 Pine Street; Harrisburg, PA 17101; 717-783-7142; www.dos.state.pa.us/bpoa/nurbd/mainpage.htm

Commonwealth of Puerto Rico Board of Nurse Examiners; 800 Roberto H. Todd Avenue; Room 202, Stop 18; Santurce, PR 00908; 787-725-8161

Rhode Island Board of Nurse Registration and Nursing Education; 105 Cannon Building; Three Capitol Hill; Providence, RI 02908; 401-222-5700; www.health.state.ri.us

South Carolina State Board of Nursing; 110 Centerview Drive, Suite 202; Columbia, SC 29210; 803-896-4550; www.llr.state.sc.us/pol/nursing

South Dakota Board of Nursing; 4300 South Louise Avenue, Suite C-1; Sioux Falls, SD 57106-3124; 605-362-2760; www.state.sd.us/dcr/nursing/

Tennessee State Board of Nursing; 426 Fifth Avenue North; 1st Floor-Cordell Hull Building; Nashville, TN 37247; 615-532-5166; http://170.142.76.180/bmf-bin/BMFproflist.pl

Texas Board of Nurse Examiners; 333 Guadalupe, Suite 3-460; Austin, TX 78701; 512-305-7400; www.bne.state.tx.us/

Texas Board of Vocational Nurse Examiners; William P. Hobby Building, Tower 3; 333 Guadalupe Street, Suite 3-400; Austin, TX 78701; 512-305-8100; www.bvne.state.tx.us/

Utah State Board of Nursing; Heber M. Wells Building, 4th Floor; 160 East 300 South; Salt Lake City, UT 84111; 801-530-6628; www.commerce.state.ut.us/

Vermont State Board of Nursing; 109 State Street; Montpelier, VT 05609-1106; 802-828-2396; http://vtprofessionals.org/nurses/

Virgin Islands Board of Nurse Licensure; Veterans Drive Station; St. Thomas, VI 00803; 340-776-7397

Virginia Board of Nursing; 6606 West Broad Street, 4th Floor; Richmond, VA 23230; 804-662-9909; www.dhp.state.va.us/

Washington State Nursing Care Quality Assurance Commission; Department of Health; 1300 Quince Street SE; Olympia, WA 98504-7864; 360-236-4740; www.doh.wa.gov/nursing/

West Virginia Board of Examiners for Licensed Practical Nurses; 101 Dee Drive; Charleston, WV 25311; 304-558-3572; www.lpnboard.state.wv.us/

West Virginia Board of Examiners for Registered Professional Nurses; 101 Dee Drive; Charleston, WV 25311; 304-558-3596; www.state.wv.us/nurses/rn/

Wisconsin Department of Regulation and Licensing; 1400 East Washington Avenue; P.O. Box 8935; Madison, WI 53708; 608-266-0145; www.drl.state.wi.us/

Wyoming State Board of Nursing; 2020 Carey Avenue, Suite 110; Cheyenne, WY 82002; 307-777-7601; http://nursing.state.wy.us/

Reprinted by permission of the National Council of State Boards of Nursing, Inc., Chicago, IL from the NCSBN Web site www.ncsbn.org

Abbreviations and Acronyms

AD	Associate Degree
ADN	Associate Degree Nurse (nursing)
AIDS	acquired immunodeficiency syndrome
ATT	authorization to test
BA	Bachelor of Arts
BP	blood pressure
BSN	Bachelor of Science in Nursing
CAT	computerized adaptive testing
CD-ROM	computer disk read-only memory
CNA	certified nurse assistant
CPR	cardiopulmonary resuscitation
GPA	grade point average
LPN	licensed practical nurse
LP/VN	licensed practical/vocational nurse
LVN	licensed vocational nurse
NCLEX®	National Council Licensure Examination
NCLEX-PN®	National Council Licensure Examination–Practical Nurse
NCLEX-RN®	National Council Licensure Examination–Registered Nurse
NCSBN	National Council of State Boards of Nursing
NFLPN	National Federation of Licensed Practical Nurses
NP	nurse practitioner
PhD	Doctor of Philosophy
RN	registered nurse
UAP	unlicensed assistive personnel

Answers to Review Questions

CHAPTER 1

1. c
2. a
3. c

CHAPTER 2

1. d
2. c
3. a
4. b

CHAPTER 3

1. a
2. b
3. a

CHAPTER 4

1. d
2. c
3. c
4. a
5. b

GLOSSARY

accountability   Responsibility for actions and inactions performed by oneself or others.

assertiveness   A way of expressing oneself without insulting others.

assignment   Term frequently used to describe the transfer of activities from one person to another; involves the downward or lateral transfer of both responsibility and accountability for an activity.

autocratic   Task-oriented leadership style based on the premise that the leader knows best.

competencies   Specific skills or tasks (e.g., blood glucose monitoring) needed for a particular position.

computerized adaptive testing (CAT)   A methodology for determining, by computer, a candidate's competence in the subject for which the candidate is being tested.

conflict   A clash, competition, or mutual interference of opposing forces or qualities (e.g., ideas, interests) that can be severe (sharp disagreement or fighting) or mild (subtle or unconscious opposition to an idea or action).

confrontation   The act of facing an unpleasant situation or a person who has opposing views.

cover letter   A letter to accompany a résumé that introduces you and your résumé for the purpose of getting a potential employer to read your résumé.

delegation   Process of transferring to a competent individual the authority to perform a specific task in a specific situation.

democratic   Leadership style in which every member of the team is asked for input.

evaluation   The act of examining and judging the quality and degree to which a person performs expected duties.

job description   A written outline of job responsibilities.

laissez-faire   A passive, nondirect approach that gives leadership responsibilities to the group rather than to one person.

leadership   The ability to influence or motivate others to set and achieve goals.

management   Accomplishment of tasks through the effective use of people and resources.

National Council Licensure Examination (NCLEX)®   An examination developed by the National Council of State Boards of Nursing that boards of nursing use in their licensure decision making; the NCLEX-PN® is given to LP/VN candidates, and the NCLEX-RN® is given to RN candidates.

organizational chart   A visual representation of the relationship of one department to another within a facility or the relationship of the facility to other facilities in a health care network.

participative   A mix of autocratic and democratic leadership styles in which the leader makes proposals to the group, invites group criticism and comments, and then uses the feedback to make the final decision.

policy   A written description of an employer's expectations for handling various situations.

procedure   Step-by-step instructions describing the processes for performing various tasks.

reference   People, such as colleagues, instructors, or employers, who can verify and support your professional and educational background claims.

résumé   A job-hunting tool that summarizes employment qualifications.

situational   Leadership style that depends on the situation, that is, the circumstances and people involved.

time management   A technique to help individuals get thing done efficiently and effectively.

INDEX

Note: Page numbers in **bold type** reference tables and figures.